ALLIES OR ADVERSARIES

Revitalizing the Medical Staff Organization

ALLIES OR ADVERSARIES

Revitalizing the Medical Staff
Organization

Craig E. Holm

ACHE Management Series

Health Administration Press

Your board, staff, or clients may also benefit from this book's insight. For more information on quantity discounts, contact the Health Administration Press Marketing Manager at (312) 424-9470.

08   07   06   05   04   5   4   3   2   1

Library of Congress Cataloging-in-Publication Data

Holm, Craig E., 1954–
    Allies or adversaries: revitalizing the medical staff organization/ Craig E. Holm.
        p ; cm.
    Includes bibliographical references.
    ISBN 1-56793-223-1 (alk. paper)
       1. Hospital-physician relations—United States. 2. Hospitals—Medical staff—
    United States. 3. Health facilities—United States—Personnel management. I. Title.
       [DNLM: 1. Hospital-Physician Relations—United States. 2. Medical Staff,
    Hospital—organization & administration—United States. 3. Personnel
    Administration, Hospital—methods—United States. WX 150 H747a 2004]
    RA971.9.H648 2004
    32.1'1'0683—dc22

                                                              20040472375

The paper used in this publication meets the minimum requirements of American National Standard for Information Sciences—Permanence of Paper for Printed Library Materials, ANSI Z39.48-1984. ⊚ ™

Acquisitions manager: Audrey Kaufman; project manager: Joyce Sherman; layout editor: Amanda J. Karvelaitis; cover designer: Betsy Pérez.

Health Administration Press
A division of the Foundation of the
American College of Healthcare Executives
1 North Franklin Street, Suite 1700
Chicago, IL 60606-4425
(312) 424-2800

Contents

Foreword

"But let it not be thought for one moment that the pinnacle of hospital evolution has been reached or that the final page of its colorful history has been written. Just so long as there remains in this world a humanitarian impulse, just so long as man feels compassion, love, and sympathy for his neighbor will there be hospitals. In the past hospitals have changed as conditions have changed. In the future they will continue to change to meet the additional demands of their communities."

—*Malcolm T. MacEachern, M.D.,*
Hospital Organization and Management, *1940 edition*

NEARLY 100 YEARS ago, a period of remarkable reform in United States healthcare got underway. In 1910, educator Abraham Flexner, under sponsorship of the Carnegie Foundation, published his landmark report, *Medical Education in the United States and Canada.* This comprehensive report examined all purported medical schools in the United States and Canada. More importantly, it signified the end of the diploma mill facilities then extant and firmly enshrined the Johns Hopkins medical education model that had been developed in Baltimore by Sir William Osler and colleagues during the late nineteenth century. Just three years later, on May 5, 1913, the American College of Surgeons was organized in Washington, DC. As stated in a subsequent document (ACS 1935),

The College is concerned fundamentally with matters of character and of training, with the betterment of hospitals and of teaching facilities in medical schools and hospitals, with laws which relate to medical practice and privilege, and with an unselfish protection of the public from incompetent medical service.

The early work of the College culminated in 1918 with the creation of its Hospital Standardization Program (HSP). The purpose of this program was to promote the work of the College, as quoted above, through the promulgation of a minimum standard for hospitals throughout the United States and Canada. This minimum standard encompassed five substandards, the first of which was "That physicians and surgeons privileged to practice in the hospital be organized as a definite group or staff. . . . The word *staff* is here defined as the group of doctors who practice in the hospital" (ACS 1935).

Thus was born the hospital medical staff organization, an entity that has survived structurally intact as a quasi-independent body within the overall organizational structure of the hospital. Despite the increasing complexity of healthcare; the growing sophistication of treatment, and thus increasing physician political power; and the transformation of medical practice into a relatively high income profession, a common interest held medical staffs to their hospitals throughout much of the twentieth century: each was dependent on the other for its existence and economic well-being, and an unquestioning public continued to reward both physicians and hospitals for ever "doing more."

Perhaps the beginning of the end of the largely symbiotic relationship between hospitals and their medical staffs occurred in 1982, when Medicare began funding hospital care on a case-based pricing method, using diagnosis-related groups, which no longer paid hospitals essentially on their costs. At the same time, however, Medicare kept physicians on a pure fee-for-service payment basis. Suddenly, hospitals could benefit by utilization review aimed at reducing the cost of care, while physicians continued to earn more by doing ever more. Thus, an economic wedge was created between hospitals and their medical staff physicians. Now, for the first time in history, physicians doing more (and thus earning more) in their hospital practices no longer necessarily benefited the hospital. In fact, excessive physician-ordered utilization could now cause financial harm to hospitals. Particularly in smaller facilities, a few high-utilization physicians might bankrupt the hospital. The historical symbiosis between hospitals and their medical staffs was over.

While tensions between hospitals and physicians resulting from these misaligned financial incentives grew during the late 1980s, the true disintegration of the symbiotic social contract between physicians and hospitals came to fruition under the pressures that aggressive managed care entities were able to exert as the 1990s proceeded. As Paul Starr, Pulitzer Prize–winning author of *The Social Transformation of American Medicine*, declared in a 1990 speech, "No matter how dramatically you think healthcare has changed in the last decade, now is the time before the revolution. Year by year, the existing system is coming unstuck" (Modern Healthcare 1990). As this book demonstrates, Starr was prescient.

Craig Holm, CHE, and his coauthors offer a comprehensive and well-reasoned description of just how the historical bond between hospitals and their medical staffs "came unstuck" under the vastly changed economic pressures of the 1990s. Indeed, they declare boldly and accurately right at the beginning of Chapter 1 that, as of today, "Medical staff organizations, as the overseer of the fundamental relationship between hospitals and physicians, are an endangered species in the healthcare world." Based on my work in the1990s and my post-millennium experience working with hospitals all over the United States, I agree wholly with this assessment of the current state of hospital–medical staff relationships. As of today, the historical symbiosis is gone. In its place, we now see the following:

- Physicians who increasingly curtail, even abandon, their hospital practices under cost/revenue pressures, forcing them to concentrate on their office practices
- A generation of physicians who are more attuned to lifestyle and family values, and thus less interested in the collegial

medical staff culture that derived from the earlier eras of HSP and the Joint Commission on Accreditation of Healthcare Organizations and served as a form of social glue between hospitals and physicians

- A resulting smaller pool of physicians and an increasing militancy of physicians reluctant to provide emergency services specialty coverage and, additionally, often demanding payment for work that previously was considered part of the territory of medical staff membership

- Physicians finding that, as the inexorable trend to outpatient medicine continues, their economic self-interest leads them to seek revenue streams formerly within the hospital's domain, and vice versa. In some cases, this economic competition gives way to open warfare, as, for example, a powerful cardiology group builds its own ambulatory heart center, using the hospital only for its most difficult (and possibly inadequately reimbursed) cases, and the hospital opens a diabetes clinic, thus competing with every internist and perhaps the pediatricians on its medical staff.

- Blatant economic credentialing, that is, hospitals removing physician investors in competing enterprises, such as an ambulatory surgicenter, from their medical staffs

- Lawsuits being brought between hospitals and physicians, as traditional values that have tied physicians to hospitals yield to the economic pressures each group faces.

This is where this book makes a unique and important contribution. It offers in-depth analysis regarding the dynamics underlying hospital–medical staff dysfunction that is now epidemic in the United States. The book further provides comprehensively thought-out approaches to all leaders, both physician and administrative, who must deal with elements of this dysfunction on a daily basis. It thus offers to medical staffs a plausible and workable pathway back, as Chapter 1 suggests, from "near extinction to relevancy."

Chapter by chapter, Holm and his colleagues explore the current major influences affecting medical staff organizations. Chapter 2 includes ten on-target trends identified by the late, highly respected healthcare futurist, Russ Coile.

Hugo Finarelli, in Chapter 3, offers important information and invaluable guidance on the use of medical staff development planning as a method of both rationalizing the physician supply issue for all types of hospitals and building new relationships with physician members of the medical staff.

Chapters 4 and 5 address the misalignment of incentives that has come to plague current hospital–medical staff relations. The focus of Chapter 4 is on incentives that might foster physician "loyalty," and Chapter 5 discusses competitive strategies that might embrace and integrate physicians into collaborative hospital-physician enterprises. Given the powerful pull of economic forces that are now splitting physicians from hospitals, this aspect of the book is particularly germane to today's hospital leaders, both clinical and non-clinical. Holm and his coworkers do not shrink from the tough realities of some medical markets. This book offers tough advice, for both physicians and administrators, on implementing strategies in markets where collaboration proves unworkable and thus leaders must make decisions based on hard-nosed competitive factors.

In the end, however, Holm holds out greatest promise for those who wish to build effective new working relationships with today's physicians, specifically with those who might form the core of the future hospital–medical staff organization. He thus offers in Chapter 6 well-considered practical approaches for those who favor collaboration over competition in the higher service of community health needs, as opposed to narrowly defined provider (economic) interest.

Finally, in its closing chapter, this book offers an extraordinarily useful schema depicting a spectrum of possible hospital-physician relationships, along with explicit guidelines and criteria that might guide prospective relationships. It is a capstone chapter, offering readers specific direction on how to pull together prior information into an action plan for engaging physicians and creating the future hospital–medical staff organization.

The book is replete with actual examples of innovative initiatives through which many forward-thinking healthcare leaders are already lighting pathways to improved hospital-physician relationships. In fact, some larger trends may already be naturally facilitating such improved relationships. For example, the withdrawal of large numbers of physicians from treating their hospitalized patients, together with the concomitant rise of the hospitalist/intensivist (fueled further by encouragement from such quarters as the Leapfrog Group), is already having the observable effect of reestablishing a core group of physicians who are hospital based and whose destinies are far more naturally aligned with those of their hospitals than today's independently practicing physicians. I agree with the author's prediction that the successful hospital of the future will feature a relatively smaller number of physicians practicing nearly exclusively at the facility, with both professional and economic incentives fully aligned with that of the institution. Such a hospital would indeed be a formidable competitor—perhaps one that might someday put an end to an era many of us perceive as destructive because of competitive behaviors that have arisen in so many U.S. communities today.

Perhaps major reform in U.S. healthcare runs in 100-year cycles. Let us hope so. Virtually all stakeholders (and who is not a healthcare stakeholder?) now agree that our healthcare system is, nearly 100 years after the Flexner report, in dire need of reform. This work offers invaluable guidance to both clinical and nonclinical leaders wishing to steer their institution out of today's preoccupation with survival, economic scarcity, and sometimes cutthroat provider competition. It highlights a reemergent focus on professional and institutional growth and development in the service of community and societal benefit—that is, toward genuine healthcare reform. Perhaps today's leaders, armed with the valuable information assembled in this book, might just create new energy for the American College of Surgeons' original 1913 vision of "direct advantage to all society because of [ACS's] definite aim to benefit the public through improved hospitalization."

—Martin D. Merry, M.D.
Adjunct Associate Clinical Professor of
Health Management and Policy,
University of New Hampshire, and
Senior Advisor for Medical Affairs,
New Hampshire Hospital Association and
Foundation for Healthy Communities

REFERENCES

American College of Surgeons. 1935. *Yearbook*, 22nd ed. Chicago: American College of Surgeons.

Flexner. A. 1910. *Medical Education in the United States and Canada. A Report to the Carnegie Foundation for the Advancement of Teaching*. New York: Carnegie Foundation.

MacEachern, M. T. 1940. *Hospital Organization and Management*. Chicago: Physicians' Record Co.

Modern Healthcare. 1990. "Quotable." Paul Starr quote. *Modern Healthcare* March 26: 58.

Preface

THE TITLE FOR this book, *Allies or Adversaries: Revitalizing the Medical Staff Organization*, was not selected until after the book had been written. When my publisher suggested it as an alternative to the original working title *The Medical Staff of the Future*, I was sold. As we look to the future, hospitals, systems, and physicians have a fundamental critical choice: Will they be allies or adversaries? And if they choose to be allies, what vehicle or forum will be used to ensure that collaboration truly occurs? I believe our best opportunities for collaboration lie with medical staff organizations rather than newly created, independent organizations.

Without a doubt, medical staff organizations have been allowed to languish into near uselessness in many hospitals and systems, often existing merely as a credentialing and accrediting body or as a reason to meet the committee and meeting requirements of accreditation and licensure organizations. In few situations have physicians earned or been granted substantive input into the management and direction of hospitals and systems through the medical staff organization or by any other means.

But the medical staff structure has enormous potential. It provides a forum for quality-of-care issues and clinical care questions and concerns. Medical staff department meetings and full medical staff organization meetings provide a periodic forum for physicians to interact with their colleagues and for hospital leaders to gain insight into physician concerns and initiate resolution.

We are truly at a crossroads for physician-hospital relationships. The dust is settling after the failed efforts in the late 1980s and 1990s to integrate, or some might say bind, physicians to hospitals and systems. Physicians have responded by pursuing initiatives that place them in direct competition with hospitals. Add to this the fact that many physicians work exclusively in the office or outpatient setting, sometimes with the help of hospitalists, and require little, if any, contact or interaction with an acute-care facility. It is overwhelmingly apparent that many physicians no longer want or need to participate in a medical staff organization. That said, some evidence indicates that significant collaboration is occurring between medical staffs and hospitals and systems through the formation of economic joint ventures, affiliated physician groups (sometimes in employment relationships or other relationships; these are discussed more fully in Chapter 4), and other creative arrangements.

The burden will be on the shoulders of hospital and system leaders to create a medical staff organization that will help them compete more effectively in a market in which competition with traditional acute-care providers shows no signs of abating. Hospital leaders must explore approaches for working collegially with physicians, regaining lost trust, and promoting active involvement in the medical staff organization. Patience, perseverance, a commitment of resources, and a willingness to truly listen to physician concerns and ideas will help ensure that medical staff organizations are revitalized into meaningful entities that help drive the success of hospitals and systems.

Physicians who choose to be allies with hospitals and systems should be rewarded with partnership opportunities that provide true value. When being allies is no longer an option, hospitals and systems must weigh the risks and rewards of pursuing competitive strategies in partnership with aligned physicians to thwart physician initiatives that threaten hospitals' market position, financial performance, and ability to be a full-service community resource.

The stakes are high. The ability of hospitals and systems to provide quality healthcare services in partnership with private practice, community-based physicians is in jeopardy. Will everyone pick a different corner of the ring and come out fighting, wasting community resources in their battle for survival and a share of the shrinking healthcare expenditure pie? Or will reason prevail and opportunities be seized so that patients, physicians, and hospitals are all winners? The choice is yours. Hopefully, this book will provide food for thought as more meaningful and constructive relationships between hospitals and staff physicians are debated and implemented.

Acknowledgments

WHEN I WROTE my first book, *Next Generation Physician–Health System Partnerships*, in 2000, I believed that the general relationship between hospitals and systems and physicians was at an all-time low based on what I had observed in my 25 years working in healthcare. In that book, I describe ways to improve physician-hospital relationships. However, in retrospect, I realize that while I acknowledged that the environment created for developing partnerships was important, too much emphasis was placed on the actual organizational models or structures. I have learned since that it is not about the model, but what the model does. This book focuses on what the model does and should do.

In writing this book, I interviewed more than 50 healthcare leaders, including physician executives, private practice physicians, hospital administrators, and department managers. Success stories were rare, so I felt compelled to interview more people. One of those people was the late Russell C. Coile, Jr., a renowned healthcare futurist who passed away in 2003. Russ predicted that successful hospitals are those that put high octane into partnerships with physicians, which supports the concept I mentioned above—that what the partnership does is important. In Russ' research about the hospital of the future, he was adamant about the pursuit of quality, operational efficiency, and other competitive attributes. This book focuses on the medical staff organization's role in the overall partnership between hospitals and their aligned physicians as they prepare for the future together.

Several people were particularly helpful in converting this book from concept to reality. Russ Coile and Alan Zuckerman provided insight and served as thought leaders; Hugo Finarelli was invaluable with his Chapter 3 contribution, which details the analytically rigorous process he developed for medical staff development planning. Thanks to the many healthcare leaders quoted in this book for their contributions to this topic. Shraddha Patel, one of our staff analysts, helped research many of the ideas in this book. Susan Arnold contributed her insights, organization, and superlative editorial skills. Thanks, Dad, for telling me I couldn't come to your lake house until the book draft was done. My kids, Shannon, Spencer, and Connor, tolerated me going upstairs to my office weeknights and weekends to work on this. And a special thanks to my wife, Kare, for challenging me to strive in this profession. Perhaps on our 25th anniversary in 2005, the Phillies will actually win the World Series again, as they did during our honeymoon.

CHAPTER 1

From Near Extinction
to Relevancy

Craig E. Holm and Richard Afable

MEDICAL STAFF ORGANIZATIONS, which serve as the fundamental relationship between hospitals and physicians, are an endangered species in the healthcare world. The troubles facing medical staff organizations have the potential to be as detrimental as the unwelcome change inflicted on hospitals and medical staffs by managed care. In the early 1990s the managed care invasion prompted futurists to predict, "Just as the railways faded into bit players in the last century, so hospitals will fade in the next" (Morrison 1994). Granted, the predictions of Morrison and others about the impact of managed care never fully materialized. But managed care has had far-reaching and substantial effects on healthcare delivery, including causing hospital closures, dwindling operating margins, and the sale of not-for-profit entities to for-profit management companies.

In a similar manner, the challenges facing physicians, hospitals, and systems could essentially render the traditional medical staff organization model obsolete and ineffective. The medical staff organization's role of fostering some degree of alignment between hospitals and physicians may soon be a relic of a bygone era. If medical staff organizations are relegated to a minor role, healthcare organizations will have lost one of the hallmarks of their mission: the ability to provide healthcare services to their community in partnership with physicians.

LOOKING BACK

Historically, a hospital's medical staff organization has been the forum through which the physicians practicing at a hospital are granted credentials and privileges. The medical staff organization also serves as the formal, legal body necessary to meet Joint Commission on Accreditation of Healthcare Organizations (Joint Commission) requirements for accreditation, state licensure, and quality oversight.

In theory, medical staff organizations are also vehicles that allow physicians to have input into the workings of the healthcare organization, including planning, service development, budget development, and clinical quality. But in far too many institutions, the medical staff organization has been relegated to serving merely as a mandated entity to fulfill the credentialing and accreditation requirements.*

Opportunities for physicians to have substantive and meaningful input into the life of the healthcare organization have been rare. Medical staff leadership positions are often assigned to senior, retiring, emeritus physicians instead of young, entrepreneurial physicians who may challenge status quo initiatives and plans. Even as the relationships of physicians to hospitals and systems have undergone massive change and realignment—employment and acquisition models, independent practice associations, physician-hospital organizations, management service organizations, independent provider organizations, foundation models, staff models, and physician

---

*It is important to note that this book is not about the role and function of the medical staff as a legal entity to meet Joint Commission requirements.

practice management companies—the role and function of the medical staff organization has remained largely static.

POWERFUL FORCES AT WORK

A host of emerging trends is now threatening the relevancy of the traditional medical staff organization role and function.

Competitive Initiatives

Physician initiatives such as freestanding imaging centers, ambulatory surgery centers, and independent specialty hospitals place physicians in direct competition with hospitals and health systems. Hospital responses to physician-led competition have ranged from ignoring the potential damage to their market position and financial performance to much harsher stances. Some organizations are terminating or restricting medical staff credentials and denying physicians access to hospital facilities if they pursue competitive initiatives. To date, most courts have sided with hospitals that have restricted privileges or medical staff membership, although these hardball tactics must be pursued carefully, as prevailing laws view competition as beneficial.

Office-Based Physicians Independent of the Hospital

Increasingly, many physicians work exclusively in the office or outpatient setting and require little, if any, contact or interaction with an acute care facility. Common examples are office-based primary care physicians supported by hospitalists, ophthalmologists, dermatologists, allergists, rheumatologists, and other subspecialists. With hospitalists emerging as an increasingly viable option to support the hospital workload of practitioners, more and more physicians are finding that they no longer need to step foot inside any acute-care facility.

Failure of Most Economic Integration Efforts

The mantra for the integration of physicians with hospitals in the late 1980s and 1990s was primary care practice acquisition and employment. These primary care physicians were often viewed as feeder networks of capitated lives in a gatekeeper model of health-care delivery under managed care. In this model, capitation means that a specified amount of money is prepaid for a particular set of services. Gatekeepers are primary care physicians in HMOs or PPOs who directly provide care and authorize or request authorization for medical services they do not provide.

Since the gatekeepers were often employees of hospitals or systems, this model is an example of full economic integration of hospitals with physicians. But for the vast majority of the country, and especially east of the Rocky Mountains, the gatekeeper model and capitation as a dominant payment system never caught on as many anticipated it would.

According to Robert Kazel (2003), "deciding it's not worth ticking off physicians and patients for a system that's not saving any money, some health plans are dropping the so-called gatekeeper model that has been a bulwark of managed care." Anthem Blue Cross and Blue Shield eliminated most referral requirements for its HMO patients (some 400,000 members) in Indiana, Kentucky, and Ohio in January 2003. Blue Cross of California now allows its medical groups to have patients go directly to certain specialists such as allergists, dermatologists, and otolaryngologists (Kazel 2003).

Of note is that this emerging rejection of the gatekeeper model by physicians and consumers alike is contrary to the increases in the gatekeeper model cited several years ago. The Center for Studying Health System Change reported that the average percentage of patients for whom their primary care physician served as a gatekeeper increased to 44.6 percent in 2001 from 41 percent in 1997 (Kazel 2003). The percentage of physicians serving as a gatekeeper for at least half of their patients also went up to 36.9 percent in 2001 from 31.7 percent in 1997 (Kazel 2003). But as the late Russell C. Coile, Jr., a healthcare futurist, suggested, "this data may represent the high point for the gatekeeper relationship" (Coile 2003).

National trends are indicating less capitation and less managed care. The Medical Group Management Association (MGMA) reports that the median percentage of capitation revenue fell from 15.6 percent in 1998 to 10.9 percent in 1999 for multispecialty groups with capitation revenues (Redling 2001). A national survey of 300 hospitals and physician groups found that 31 percent of hospitals were using capitation in 2001, down from 46 percent in 2000 (Benko 2002). This pronounced trend toward less capitation and managed care and deemphasis of the primary care provider-gatekeeper model has put the power of choice into consumers' hands. Patients are increasingly able to self-refer, meaning that hospitals, systems, and affiliated subspecialists no longer have a guaranteed source of referrals from owned primary care practices and employed primary care physicians as they did in the 1980s and 1990s.

SAME STRUCTURE, DIFFERENT ROLE

The existing, traditional medical staff organization structure has in many ways served hospitals and physicians well. The medical staff organization provides a forum for attending to quality-of-care issues and initiatives, individual practitioner credentialing, and other areas of clinical importance. Further, periodic medical staff department and overall staff meetings and functions provide a formal forum for physicians to interact with other colleagues and hospital leaders. The medical staff organization holds some value, albeit diminishing as perceived by physician members.

Instead of starting from scratch and creating a new medical staff organization structure, healthcare organizations should direct their focus on creating a new role, culture, and set of responsibilities for their medical staff organization. A helpful framework for rethinking medical staff organizations is to consider that they should be characterized as the relationship *with* physicians, rather than the organization *for* physicians. Hospitals and systems must create new relationships with physicians, using the medical staff organization to meet the changing needs of physicians and healthcare organizations.

In some cases medical staff organizations will be the key vehicle for integration of physicians and healthcare organizations. In other instances they will help physicians and healthcare organizations compete more effectively in an increasingly competitive healthcare market.

Physicians could be categorized as either adversaries or allies with a healthcare organization. This book will discuss different strategies to be employed based on these categorizations. If physicians are potential or likely allies, then hospitals and systems should carefully evaluate partnership options, as discussed in Chapter 4. When physicians chose to take a competitive stance as adversaries, healthcare organizations must consider pursuing strategies, in partnership with aligned physicians, to secure their market position and financial performance, as reviewed in Chapter 5. Only then can hospitals and systems effectively compete head-to-head with independent physician practices.

Clearly the message is that healthcare organizations must be much more attentive to their medical staff organizations, dedicating resources to ensure that this entity vital to the well-being of hospitals, systems, and physicians is not allowed to become irrelevant. Those who choose to let their medical staff organizations languish as an insignificant and unimportant organization that merely fulfills regulatory requirements and wields little power or influence may find that the very foundation of their healthcare delivery system is eroded. In many cases private practice initiatives flourish at the expense of the traditional medical staff and their host hospital or system.

Characteristics and Functions: What Will It Look Like?

If change for medical staff organizations is necessary, then it is critical to have some vision of what a vibrant, mutually beneficial medical staff organization should look like and how it should function. The successful medical staff organization of the future should do the following:

- Create value for physician members and the sponsoring hospital or system
- Provide incentives for active membership and participation through alignment of physician and hospital incentives
- Pursue preferred partnership arrangements with physicians
- Facilitate stable and thriving referral relationships
- Be a formidable competitor for those with competitive interests
- Foster the patient community's perception of the medical staff and healthcare organization as a unified team dedicated to providing high-quality medical care and using community healthcare resources wisely
- Successfully recruit top-notch physicians, and replenish practices when physicians depart
- Evaluate and address community needs, as defined by a medical staff development plan
- Enable physicians and hospitals to garner market-competitive earnings compared to entities that contract independently

Daunting Challenges Ahead

Descriptions of how a future-oriented medical staff organization will look and function may seem simplistic when described in a neat and tidy list. But in the real world, a number of complex questions must be answered and many arduous tasks completed to transform a potential dinosaur into a new, robust entity.

- What specific adaptations to the traditional relationship with their medical staffs will hospitals and systems make to address successfully the threat posed by competing physicians?
- How do hospitals and systems cope with the increasing numbers of physicians working exclusively in their offices with little or no need to interact with hospitals?
- How do hospitals and systems and their medical staffs cope with a decline in employment of physicians? How do free-standing community hospitals with loosely aligned, independent physicians create incentives for close physician alignment?
- How do healthcare organizations manage the loss of patient "steerage" through gatekeeper referrals from employed primary care physicians working in hospital-owned practices?
- How should physicians be included in a more meaningful and effective manner in the governance and decision making for the hospital and medical staff?

This book explores strategies that will help hospitals and medical staff organizations answer these questions and create vital and strong medical staff relationships that are poised for success in an environment where competition and alienation show no signs of abating.

REFERENCES

Benko, L. 2002. "No More Risky Business." *Modern Healthcare* 32 (31): 20.

Coile. R. C., Jr. 2003. Personal interview, May 4.

Kazel. R. 2003. "Managed Care Easing Gatekeeper Hassles." *American Medical News* 46 (3): 1.

Morrison. J. I. 1994. "Railways of the Nineties." *Healthcare Forum* 37 (2): 30.

Redling, B. 2001. "Declines in Capitation Revenue Challenge Many Groups." *MGM Update* 40 (7).

CHAPTER 2

Trends Affecting Medical Staff Organizations

Craig E. Holm and Russell C. Coile, Jr.

RELATIONSHIPS BETWEEN PHYSICIANS and healthcare organizations are being influenced by a number of trends in the healthcare industry. Some of these influences are predictable; others are largely a result of factors external to hospitals and physicians. Overall, these trends have led, at a minimum, to general separation of healthcare organizations and physicians. In many cases, strained and acrimonious relationships have become all too pervasive. Using the same failed approaches will only foster further alienation.

According to Donald Zismer (2002), "The good news ... is that most groups of physicians prefer to work with the hospital. The bad news is that many hospitals turn a deaf ear to the physicians or drag the process out so long that they defect to a promoter—like MedCath. Or they do their own thing." In the not-too-distant past, physicians and hospitals at least operated in a common environment; there were few cases of head-to-head competition between physicians and hospitals. Today, the degree of separation and independence is at an all-time high.

THE TOP TEN TRENDS INFLUENCING MEDICAL STAFF ORGANIZATIONS

1. Predominance of Independent Physician Practices

The vast majority of physicians are mostly independent of, rather than integrated with, hospitals, healthcare systems, and other entities, despite the flurry of efforts in the 1990s to force physicians to integrate with specific providers. In most markets, opportunities abound to align physicians through more effective and relevant medical staff organizations. Data from the American Medical Association indicate that in 2001, 23 percent of physicians were in a solo practice environment, while nearly 37 percent of physicians practiced in self-employed groups (AMA 2003).

Physician alignment with providers other than hospital and healthcare system entities has not met with great success either. For example, physician participation in first-generation physician practice management companies (PPMCs) resulted in promises to physicians that failed to materialize. PPMCs are ultimately responsible to their parent company, whose mission historically was to create financially successful Wall Street investments, as measured in returns on stockholder shares. The inherent need of PPMCs to focus on financials, such as revenue growth and incremental earnings, set many PPMCs at odds with physicians, whose goal was to provide high-quality care in a cost-effective manner. Second-generation PPMCs, such as HealthSouth and MedCath, may be compelled to cede a portion of facility revenues to make their offerings more attractive to physicians as physicians become more savvy about the aggressive nature of PPMCs (Burns and Wholey 2000).

Hospitals and health systems may be the physicians' partner by default as long as the misadventures of the past and the mistrust created can be overcome. Much fence mending will be needed to remove the skepticism most physicians feel toward hospitals and health systems. In the words of a physician in a leadership position of a New England medical staff, "The hospital as currently structured is an inefficient and wasteful dinosaur—why should we align?" Another physician commented, "Except for big surgical cases, and the ICU and ED, physicians not only do not, but should not need the hospital."

Most physicians have chosen to remain independent of hospitals, only reluctantly participate in the membership requirements of a medical staff organization, and do little else as far as involvement in a hospital is concerned. Some physicians have followed the allure of other nimble, alternative outside partners such as for-profit ambulatory surgery centers or specialty niche hospitals. Unfortunately, many hospitals and healthcare systems offer few incentives for even a minimum level of involvement in a medical staff organization and often ignore opportunities for substantial physician alignment or involvement with a hospital.

This situation is being exacerbated by the use of hospitalists, who enable some physicians to minimize and even avoid all contact with inpatient facilities and save money in the process. A study by Robert Wachter, M.D., the physician who coined the term *hospitalist* in 1996, revealed that primary care physicians can save up to $40,000 annually by referring to hospitalists and exchanging commuting time for office time (Adams 2002).

2. Constrained Reimbursement

The 1997 Balanced Budget Act (BBA) legislation substantially reduced payments to hospitals and systems, with the most significant effects occurring in 1998 and beyond. As a result, hospital and health systems' ability to take on additional capital investments for initiatives such as practice acquisition and economic joint ventures has been largely eroded. Some pundits, like Ken Mack (2002), believe that these types of investments are necessary even with limited capital; however, for many hospitals and health systems, the focus has been solely on cost cutting and practice divestiture rather than on any substantial new investment in physician-hospital relationships. From the physician perspective, according to Richard Afable, M.D., "In the absence of managed care capitation, the value of full integration of hospitals and physicians is just not there" (Afable 2003).

Medicare Part B (i.e., professional fees) fee cuts of 5.4 percent in 2002 were followed with a 1.4 percent fee increase in 2003 after a contentious battle over a proposed, potential 4.4 percent reduction for 2003. For 2004, fees were originally targeted to decline by 4.2 percent, but final congressional action resulted in another 1.5 percent increase in that year (Hawryluk 2004). These fluctuations follow the 5 percent decline in physician payments from Medicare in 2002 (Holder and Cochran 2003). Healthcare strategist Alan Zuckerman predicts that physicians may close their practices to new Medicare patients if the Centers for Medicare & Medicaid Services (CMS) continues to enact reimbursement cuts and as federal and state budget deficits are likely to continue to increase in 2004 and beyond (Zuckerman 2003).

The overall result of constrained reimbursement is that physicians are increasingly motivated to find other revenue sources, often through partnerships with others. Meanwhile, hospitals are hindered in terms of their ability to work with physicians and support practices in meaningful, financially valuable ways that require any significant capital or operating funds or in a fashion perceived to be expeditious.

3. Changes in Ambulatory Services Delivery

New technology is serving as a key driver in fostering separatism and independence among health organizations and physician practices. Technology development, along with changing reimbursement and practice patterns, have facilitated the movement of healthcare services, both inpatient and outpatient, out of the traditional hospital setting. This movement of services has tipped the scales, in many cases, in favor of entrepreneurial physicians. Declining professional fees, rising practice expenses, and the opportunity to offset declining earnings by capturing technical fees motivates physicians to develop diagnostic and treatment services in their practice.

For example, most ophthalmologic surgery is now performed in ambulatory centers independent of traditional hospital operating rooms. Many other ambulatory procedures in specialties such as otorhinolaryngology, orthopedics, general surgery, endoscopy, imaging, and physical therapy are also provided outside the traditional hospital setting.

As reported in *Futurescan 2003*, "nearly one-third of all outpatient surgery is now provided in freestanding facilities, the majority of which are owned by doctors and entrepreneurial companies" (Coile 2003, 31).

4. Elimination of Certificate-of-Need Restrictions

In many states, certificate-of-need (CON) regulations have served as a barrier to market entry for potential new developers of healthcare services, whether they be a competitor hospital, a group of physicians, or an independent (in most cases, for-profit) developer. Without CON regulations, providers of healthcare services are in a better position to compete with existing providers, as is the case in any free market environment. Even the American Hospital Association (AHA) is weighing in on the CON issue. A key thrust of the AHA 2004 advocacy agenda is "reducing the regulatory burden" (AHA 2004), which makes it seem unlikely that the association would support revitalized CON regulations.

A small physician group practice in New Hampshire illustrates how CON regulations can restrict the development of competitive facilities. In 1998, the Orthopedic Professional Association, a group of eight orthopedic surgeons, constructed a freestanding ambulatory surgery center (ASC). The ASC stood idle for over a year because of a feud with the nearby hospital. According to the administrator of the Orthopedic Professional Association, "the situation had exploded into an all-out war in the community" (Thompson 2000).

As of January 2004, 26 states still had acute-care certificate-of-need programs, and 24 states had repealed CON regulations (see Figure 2.1). The predominant trend, however, has been to repeal CON regulations and resultant restrictions or allow them to sunset (AHPA 2004a, 2004b).

Richard Afable, M.D., provides the physician perspective on CON regulation: "Freestanding ambulatory surgery centers avoid CON requirements through Stark loopholes yet to be closed. With neither CON restrictions, nor Stark prohibitions, new healthcare services can be developed in the open market. However, the trend is clearly for more, rather than less, Stark and other regulatory restrictions being enacted by the federal government. This could dramatically reduce the ability of physicians to develop independent inpatient and outpatient services" (Afable 2003).

5. Decline in Physician Professional Fees

In most specialties, physician reimbursement, paid to physicians in accordance with professional fee schedules, has stayed level or declined (Pugh 2003). Much of the struggle to keep practice revenue above operating costs is fueled by declining Medicare and Medicaid payments.

The feeling among physicians that they are working harder than ever for less pay is more than theoretical. In cardiology, higher gross charges and volumes of procedures indicate these physicians are more productive. However, according to the Medical Group Management Association (MGMA), lower reimbursement coupled with more staff and associated expenses to handle the additional volume of these harder-working cardiologists lead to lower operating income (Dunevitz 2000). Internal medicine physicians have experienced similar rises in productivity without the higher revenues typically associated with increased work. Between 1996 and 2000, while

Figure 2.1. Certificate-of-Need (CON) Programs Existing as a Barrier to Market Entry

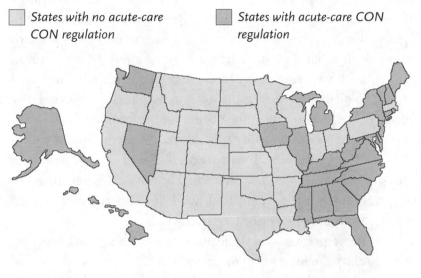

☐ *States with no acute-care CON regulation*   ☐ *States with acute-care CON regulation*

Source: Health Strategies & Solutions (2003).

this specialty's median gross charges increased 18 percent, median compensation levels only rose by six percent (MGMA 1997, 2001).

Higher productivity without associated increases in revenue is in sharp contrast to the pre–managed care era prior to the 1980s. According to University of Pennsylvania bioethics professor Glenn McGee, "Before managed care, physicians were paid more to do more, and all the fat in the healthcare system went to physician salaries—to the tune of 10 to 15 percent salary increases per year" (Stark and Gammage 2003).

Philadelphia is a prime example of physician fee schedules being hard hit by the managed care revolution. In January 2002, the Pennsylvania Medical Society (2002) released the findings from a study of health maintenance organization (HMO) payments in 25 major metropolitan areas: Philadelphia ranked the lowest in the country among these 25 major metropolitan areas. The reality is that payments from commercial HMO payers to physicians can be as low as 75 to 80 percent of the prevailing Medicare fee schedule. In sharp contrast, in other markets in the Southeast and Midwest, commercial HMO payments can be as high as 160 to 170 percent or more of the Medicare fee schedule (Health Strategies & Solutions 2003).

Prevailing fee schedules are often one important trigger for acrimonious physician-hospital relationships. As a result, physicians in markets with low reimbursement have been particularly motivated to develop diagnostic and treatment services in their practices. These initiatives attempt to offset the decline in professional fees by capturing the technical or facility fees derived by ownership of equipment and employment of staff associated with the provision of ancillary healthcare services. Alternatively, physicians may invest in real estate to earn passive income, work more hours each day, or practice for more years prior to retirement.

In many respects, much of the outmigration of ambulatory diagnostic and treatment services to physician offices can be considered an inevitable result of influences such as CON programs, technology development, and decline in professional fee schedules. *Futurescan 2003* (Coile 2003, 10) reports that gastroenterology was 81 percent hospital based in 1994, versus 64 percent hospital based in 2001. Ophthalmology was 44 percent hospital based in 1994, versus 32 percent in 2001.

However, hospitals and physicians do have some regulatory incentive to work together in the provision of ambulatory services. Specifically, Stark guidelines provide latitude for hospitals and physicians to structure joint venture arrangements to provide many outpatient services such as surgery and positron-emission tomography scans (for the time being), for real estate deals, and for other investments.

6. Increases in Physician Practice Expenses

On the expense side, the cost of providing care has increased dramatically. Skyrocketing malpractice expenses, staff expenses (especially nursing staff), and the cost of medical supplies and pharmaceuticals have had particularly detrimental effects on the expenses of physician practices. Exorbitant practice expenses are forcing some physicians to abandon medicine altogether or becoming a key determinant of where they practice. As noted in the *Wall Street Journal* (2003), "New doctors refuse to move to states such as West Virginia, Pennsylvania, and New Jersey, where malpractice insurance rates are staggering. The best and brightest and busiest doctors are the ones being forced out of practice."

The malpractice situation is of significant concern to medical residents. According to a survey by Merritt, Hawkins and Associates, 60 percent of 2003 third-year residents said that malpractice costs were causing them "significant concern" as they entered medical practice, compared to only 15 percent in the 2001 survey (Romano 2003). The medical school debt burden and paying for malpractice costs and other rising expenses are often perceived as insurmountable for the physician building or maintaining a medical practice.

Increased practice expenses are also influencing physician ties to medical staff organizations. Physicians are motivated to become more independent of hospitals since their livelihood is less dependent on the traditional practice environment and increasingly independent of the hospital.

For subspecialists, expense increases have been especially dramatic. For example, MGMA (2002) reported that median operating costs for cardiovascular-thoracic surgeons rose about 16 percent to $422,659, and support staff costs per full-time-equivalent physician increased from approximately $193,000 to $220,000.

As a result of declining professional fees and increasing expenses, physicians report that they are spending more time with patients, according to the Center for Studying Health System Change, but more physicians also are complaining that they do not have enough time for patient care (Trude 2003). The portion of a physician's working day spent on direct patient care increased to 87 percent from 81 percent between 1997 and 2001, but the percentage of physicians reporting inadequate time with patients grew from 28 percent to 34 percent.

Given the stresses physicians report in their offices, staying aligned with the traditional medical staff structure may be difficult for private practice, independent physicians, since such an alignment requires committee service and meeting attendance and places additional burdens on physician time. Some physicians feel strongly about the wasted time spent in committees. In the words of Stuart Brogadir, M.D., "The committees are time consuming and inefficient, racked with the same liability and hassle destroying physician practices. Why sign up for another hassle—for free? Some committees are necessary; some are bureaucratic nightmares. All are inefficient" (Brogadir 2003).

7. Lingering Effects of Physician-Hospital Misadventures

A multitude of "misadventures" have occurred as hospitals, health systems, and physicians have tried to forge mutually beneficial partnerships. One surgeon in the Southwest, a champion of an independent joint venture specialty niche hospital, explained, "I detest the local community hospital so much because of past misadventures that my goal is to develop this independent hospital to financially harm the existing hospital. Ultimately, my goal is to hold underwater _____ Health System's head until there are no more bubbles." From the healthcare administrator's perspective, many physicians lack an understanding or appreciation of what is required to create physician-hospital alliances, such as the business, regulatory, and political implications. As Robert Pickoff, M.D., chief medical officer of the Hunterdon Healthcare System in Flemington, New Jersey, reports, "Many physicians misunderstand the legal obstacles to joint ventures and misinterpret a hospital's reluctance to do so as arrogance" (Pickoff 2003).

The list of misadventures that have wreaked havoc with physician-hospital ties is lengthy. Payer risk assumption through negotiating capitated or other risk-bearing contracts and aggressive and wide-spread practice acquisition and employment are common examples that have been particularly fractious for hospitals and physicians. Medical practices owned by integrated delivery systems lost $89,480 per full-time-equivalent physician in 2000 (Reese 2002).

Practice acquisition and employment represent many faulty assumptions about the fundamental business model of healthcare delivery: that hospitals can manage physician practices better than physicians can (including assuming responsibility for billing and collections), that start-up practices will attain viability much sooner when overseen by hospitals, and that hospitals can eliminate ancillary services from practices (which often represent 15 to 25 percent of practice revenue) without threatening the practices' viability. Hospitals and systems typically failed to realize that previously autonomous physicians often lose their entrepreneurial motivation when they convert from private practice to employment, leading to lower productivity levels.

Practice acquisition and employment is still an appropriate strategy in some markets when a need to compete with other systems exists, if practice expenses are particularly onerous, or when other local market dynamics are present. Example markets where practice acquisition and employment are still robust strategies include south Florida; Milwaukee, Wisconsin; Rochester, New York; and portions of Texas and North Carolina.

Physician-hospital organizations (PHOs) and management service organizations (MSOs) also fueled mistrust and animosity among physicians, hospitals, and systems. In some cases, the formation of PHOs as risk-bearing entities was predicated on a particularly faulty assumption: that hospitals, physicians, and other healthcare providers could objectively and rationally allocate a shrinking pool of reimbursement from payers in a manner satisfactory to all parties, including physicians.

The formation of MSOs was also based on a significant faulty assumption: that hospital managers, operating in a bureaucratic, primarily inpatient-oriented hospital environment, could understand

and manage physician practices, functioning predominantly in an outpatient setting, more efficiently and effectively than could practice managers and physicians in an entrepreneurial environment.

Even physician-only networks, or independent practice associations (IPAs), have fallen out of favor. The number of IPAs has dropped from about 3,000 in the late 1990s to about 2,200 in 2003 (Terry 2003). Burns and Wholey (2000) summarize the current physician attitude as "anti-management and anti-organizational."

8. Recruitment Challenges

In many markets, escalating expenses (largely malpractice, nursing staff, and in some cases real estate expenses) coupled with level or declining professional fees have made recruitment of additional physician colleagues difficult, which in turn affects the replenishment cycle for the medical staff.

Physician supply projections will be discussed in detail in Chapter 3.

9. The Nursing Shortage

The ongoing nursing shortage may force more changes on America's physicians and hospitals. The research about the nursing shortage is compelling. A survey by the Harvard School of Public Health and the Henry J. Kaiser Family Foundation, reported in the *New England Journal of Medicine*, found that 53 percent of physicians and 65 percent of the public cited the shortage of nurses as a leading cause of medical errors (Blendon et al. 2002). Overall, 42 percent of the public and more than a third of U.S. doctors reported that they or their family members have experienced medical errors in the course of receiving medical care.

A study published in the *Journal of the American Medical Association* reports that more nurses at the bedside could save thousands of patient lives each year. Nurse researchers at the University of Pennsylvania determined that patients who have common surgeries in hospitals with low nurse-to-patient ratios have an up to 31 percent increased chance of dying (Aiken et al. 2003). *Health Care at the Crossroads: Strategies for Addressing the Evolving Nursing Crisis*, a report released in August 2002, reported that the Joint Commission on Accreditation of Healthcare Organizations examined 1,609 hospital reports of patient deaths and injuries since 1996 and found that low nursing staff levels were a contributing factor in 24 percent of the cases (American Association of Colleges of Nursing 2003).

Nursing school programs are beginning to report that admissions are rising again, but that solution will take years to remedy the growing crisis. Until the nursing shortage abates and hospitals and systems recognize that having too few nurses may actually cost more money given the high costs of replacing burnt-out nurses and caring for patients with poor outcomes, physicians will shoulder more of the burden to ensure that no medical errors occur with their patients.

10. Service Cooperation

Hospitals are asking their medical staffs to assist with customer service initiatives. Consumers rank physician communication as one of their highest-rated concerns. Hospitals that are concerned about the quality of the patient experience are seeking to engage physicians in quality efforts and the culture of service excellence. Today, over a dozen states give consumers an opportunity to rate their care in a report-card format. Medicare is considering asking hospitals to give consumers an opportunity to be heard on patient issues. Customer service initiatives provide many opportunities for hospitals and physicians to unite forces and empower the medical staff organization to play a lead role in improving patient care and satisfaction.

HOW THE TRENDS AFFECT MEDICAL STAFF ORGANIZATIONS

The trends discussed in this chapter will have far-reaching and lasting effects on medical staff organizations, as well as on the fundamental relationship between hospitals and aligned physician practices. Physicians were historically customers of hospitals and not competitors of them; then they became both customers and competitors. Hospitals tried to integrate with physicians by pursuing various partnerships, practice acquisition and employment, management service organizations, physician-hospital organizations, and global risk contracts, although most of these efforts failed. Now, more than ever, physicians are both customer and competitor, placing hospitals in the difficult position of trying to cater to their competitors for certain services and compete for others.

Two manifestations of the trends discussed in this chapter are now emerging: (1) weak, bitter, and even hostile physician-hospital relationships and (2) the proliferation of independent or "boutique" for-profit providers. The ongoing deterioration of the relationship between hospitals and physicians has led some to lose hope for repairing the damage, while others predict that there is nowhere to go but up, pointing to the vast opportunities for physicians, hospitals, and systems to work together to create a more viable and purposeful medical staff organization and build other strong physician alliances.

For-profit organizations, with ready access to capital, often fuel the fires of rivalry by helping locally based physicians strip ancillaries out of the hospital setting or creating for-profit ventures such as specialty hospitals and outpatient centers. In for-profit organizations, the business motivation is usually to target high-margin healthcare programs and services to maximize financial return.

The response of the hospital industry is to cry foul. Hospitals and systems claim that physicians are stripping out the most profitable services, leaving them with no margin to support the full range of services that the community expects. The battle over this area will be fought in local communities, in state legislatures and courts, and in Congress. Initiatives are already underway to expand physician anti-self-referral laws to preclude investments in specialty hospitals—something currently permitted but perhaps not contemplated by the drafters of the laws.

Many scenarios may emerge as the trends discussed in this chapter are felt full force across the nation. Hospitals and systems that are willing to acknowledge that the slippery downward slide of physician-hospital relationships must be halted will take aggressive action to ensure that their medical staff organizations and other physician relationships are strengthened and made relevant for the challenges ahead. The future viability of quality healthcare services provided in partnership with community physicians is at stake.

REFERENCES

Adams, D. 2002. "Hospitalist Practice: Could It Work for You?" [Online article; retrieved 10/27/03.] http://www.ama-assn.org/amednews/2002/11/11/prsa1111 .htm.

Afable, R. 2003. Personal interview, July 28.

Aiken L. H., S. P. Clarke, R. B. Cheung, D. M. Sloane, and J. H. Silber. 2003. "Educational Levels of Hospital Nurses and Surgical Patient Mortality." *Journal of the American Medical Association* 290 (12): 1617–23.

American Association of Colleges of Nursing. 2003. "About the Nursing Shortage." [Online article; retrieved 10/29/03.] http://www.aacn.nche.edu/Media /shortageresource.htm#impact.

American Health Planning Association. 2004a. "2004 Relative Scope and Review of Thresholds of CON Regulated Services." Compiled by T. R. Piper, January 27. Falls Church, VA: AHPA.

———. 2004b. "2004 Relative Scope and Thresholds of CON Regulation." January 23. Falls Church, VA: AHPA.

American Hospital Association. 2004. "Protecting Care Today, Investing in Tomorrow." *AHA News* 40 (4).

American Medical Association. 2003. *Physician Socioeconomic Statistics*. Chicago: AMA Press.

Blendon, R. J., C. M. DesRoches, M. Brodie, J. M. Benson, A. B. Rosen, C. Schneider, D. E. Altman, K. Zapert, M. J. Hermann, and A. E. Steffenson. 2002. "Views of Practicing Physicians and the Public on Medical Errors." *New England Journal of Medicine* 347 (24): 1933–40.

Brogadir, S. 2003. Personal interview, June 23.

Burns, L., and D. Wholey. 2000. "Responding to a Consolidated Healthcare System: Options for Physician Organizations." In *Future of Integrated Delivery Systems*, vol. 1, 261–323. St. Louis, MO: JAI/Elsevier, Inc.

Coile, R. C., Jr. 2003. *Futurescan 2003: A Forecast of Healthcare Trends 2003–2007*. Chicago: Health Administration Press.

Dunevitz, B. 2000. "Most Groups Seeing Higher Revenues for Increased Work." *MGM Update* 39 (18).

Health Strategies & Solutions, Inc. 2003. Company databases.

Holder, L., and A. Cochran 2003. "Recovering Physician Loyalty." *Healthcare Executive* 18 (2): 65.

Mack, K. 2002. "Are You Ready to Invest in Business Development?" *Healthcare Financial Management* 56 (10): 70.

Medical Group Management Association. 2002. *Cost Survey: 2002 Report Based on 2001 Data*. Englewood, CO: MGMA.

———. 2001. *Physician Compensation and Production Survey: 2001 Report Based on 2000 Data*. Englewood, CO: MGMA.

———. 1997. *Physician Compensation and Production Survey: 1997 Report Based on 1996 Data*. Englewood, CO: MGMA.

Pennsylvania Medical Society. 2002. "Comparison of HMO Operating Statistics in the 25 Largest MSAs in the U.S." [Online article; retrieved 11/1/03.] http://www.philamedsoc.org/community/Resources/PMS-HMO-MSA.pdf.

Pickoff, R. 2003. Personal interview, July 8.

Pugh, T. 2003. "Caught in Squeeze, Doctors Start Charging for More Services." *Philadelphia Inquirer*, June 2, D1, D10.

Reese, E. 2002. "IDS-Owned Practices Still Losing Money." *Healthcare Financial Management* 56 (4): 23.

Romano, M. 2003. "Poll: 24% of Residents Want Out." *Modern Healthcare* 33 (20): 3.

Stark, K., and J. Gammage. 2003. "Bitter Medicine." *Inquirer Magazine* June 29. [Online article; retrieved 1/9/04.] http://www.philly.com/mld/inquirer/news /special_packages/inquirer_magazine/features/6167529.htm.

Terry, K. 2003. "How IPAs are Changing." *Medical Economics* 80 (12): 52.

Thompson, E. 2000. "Duking It Out: Local Hospitals Fight Back as Physicians Bring on Competition with Specialty Facilities." *Modern Healthcare* (30) 29: 3.

Trude, S. 2003. *So Much to Do, So Little Time: Physician Capacity Constraints, 1997–2001.* Tracking Report No. 8. [Online report; retrieved 3/29/04.] http://www .hschange.com/CONTENT/556/.

Wall Street Journal. 2003. "Good Doctors Are Being Forced Out of Practice." *Wall Street Journal,* May 16, A9.

Zismer, D. 2002. "Not a Fad, a Joint Venture." *Healthcare Strategy Alert* November/December 1–3.

Zuckerman, A. 2003. Personal interview, June 12.

CHAPTER 3

A Guide to Medical Staff Development Planning

Hugo J. Finarelli, Jr.

MEDICAL STAFF DEVELOPMENT planning is a means to an end for many different constituencies.

- *Hospital leadership relies on the process* because it legitimizes recruiting additional physicians to increase utilization of hospital programs and services.
- *Boards of trustees call for the process* to determine community needs in their role as the stewards of community interests.
- *Medical staffs sometimes stonewall or sabotage the process* because it may result in additional competition for existing practices.
- *The Internal Revenue Service supports the process* because "objective documentation of community need" may justify hospitals offering financial assistance to physicians who help meet the community need.
- *Individual physician practices increasingly rely on the process* to answer the fundamental question, "Is there sufficient unmet demand in the community to support adding another physician to my practice?"

- *Academic medical centers (AMCs) rarely use the process* because their need for additional physician resources is often driven by research and teaching requirements, not clinical activities.

The *process* is medical staff development planning. The fundamental approach is to compare the population-based need for physicians within a community or geographic region with the available supply of physicians. In its simplest form, determining population-based need is a straightforward mathematical exercise in which the population in a given market or region is multiplied by a series of specialty-specific physician-to-population ratios, expressed in terms of the number of physicians required to serve a defined population of, for example, 100,000 persons.

SELECTING THE RIGHT PHYSICIAN-TO-POPULATION RATIOS

The straightforward mathematical exercise, however, soon becomes more complex. Selecting the appropriate physician-to-population ratios for a particular community or region is not a simple task. In fact, much disagreement has erupted in recent years as to whether the nation was facing a surplus or shortage of physicians.

One of the earliest studies that addressed physician need at a national level was the 1980 report of the Graduate Medical Education National Advisory Council (GMENAC 1980). This study was undertaken in response to concerns that U.S. medical schools were training too many physicians and, in particular, too many specialists. A series of subsequent reports published by the Council on Graduate Medical Education (COGME 1992, 1995, 1996) in the 1990s echoed the concerns that the nation was facing an oversupply of physicians and an imbalance of specialists (too many) versus generalists (too few). COGME went on to recommend that first-year residency positions in the United States be reduced by 22 percent and that half of all new medical school graduates be generalists (COGME 1999).

As managed care became more prominent in the early 1990s, publications such as the *Journal of the American Medical Association* and the *New England Journal of Medicine* published articles that forecast future physician need using physician-to-population ratios that reflected physician staffing patterns within staff-model and group-model HMOs like Kaiser Permanente (Kronick et al. 1993; Weiner 1994; Rivo and Kindig 1996; Schroeder 1996).

One of the most frequently referenced articles was Weiner's (1994) very thorough and thoughtful analysis of the expected effects of healthcare reform on physician workforce requirements. Weiner assumed that an estimated 40 to 65 percent of the U.S. population would be receiving care from integrated managed care networks or from staff- or group-model HMOs by 2000. Furthermore, Weiner assumed that physician requirements would be only 124 per 100,000 population in integrated networks and 146 per 100,000 in group- or staff-model HMOs. On the basis of these assumptions, Weiner predicted a surplus of 165,000 patient care physicians in 2000, virtually all in specialty areas.

History has proven, however, that calculations of physician need that are based on managed care–like ratios of 125 to 150 physicians per 100,000 population far understate expressed need in most markets. The managed care revolution has been replaced by a managed care backlash against stringent controls and limits on access to physician services. Thus, despite the fact that more than 200 physicians are now active in patient care per 100,000 population nationwide, physicians are in short supply in many communities. Furthermore, the predicted oversupply of specialists has never materialized. In some markets, patients must wait several weeks or months for non-emergency appointments in specialties where local shortages are most severe.

One expert, Richard A. Cooper, M.D., director of the Health Policy Institute, expressed a contrarian view several years ago (Cooper 1995). Two of Cooper's most recent analyses caution that economic and demographic trends portend a shortage of physicians nationwide, not a surplus (Cooper 2002; Cooper et al. 2002). Most health services researchers now agree. In fact, at its final meeting on September 17, 2003, COGME endorsed key elements of a report indicating an impending shortage of physicians nationwide. One of the recommendations in this report called for modest increases in enrollment levels for both undergraduate and graduate medical education (COGME 2003a, 2003b).

These changing recommendations create a great deal of uncertainty about which physician-to-population ratios to use to determine community need.

OTHER METHODOLOGICAL PITFALLS

Many other methodological pitfalls must be avoided when determining population-based need for physicians.

1. Not accounting for changing patterns of care. One example of a changing pattern of care is the surging demand for screening colonoscopies for detecting colon cancer, a trend that has significantly increased the need for gastroenterologists. Another trend is the explosive growth in invasive cardiology procedures, which has increased the need for interventional cardiologists, who spend most of their time in the cardiac catheterization laboratory. At the other end of the spectrum, the "gatekeeper" model of primary care delivery was expected to dramatically increase the need for family practitioners and general internists, but the gatekeeper concept has fallen out of favor in most markets, as patients have demanded more direct access to specialists.

2. Assuming that one set of physician-to-population ratios applies to all markets. Consider, for example, that metropolitan areas within the state of Ohio had an average of 244 physicians (active in patient care) per 100,000 population in calendar year (CY) 2000. By way of comparison, the rural portions of Ohio had only 92 physicians per 100,000. Metropolitan areas also showed striking differences, with Cleveland and Cincinnati reporting more than 300 physicians per 100,000 population, compared to fewer than 200 per 100,000 in several smaller metropolitan areas (Pasko and Seidman 2003).

While some of these differences in physician supply reflect true differences in population-based need (resulting from underlying differences in the health status or the age mix of the resident population, for example), the concentration of medical and surgical specialists in urban areas is largely attributable to other factors: having a sufficient population base to support highly specialized disciplines; having access to cutting-edge technology and highly trained staff; and being able to practice with renowned faculty in medical school settings or leading specialists in other large institutions. Thus, physician-to-population ratios must be adjusted to reflect both the demographics of the community to be served and the unique characteristics of the existing medical marketplace.

3. Failing to account for regionally specific practice patterns. A general standard for allocating the time a family medicine physician spends in patient care, according to Martin Lipsky, M.D., the chair of family medicine of Northwestern University Feinberg School of Medicine, is that 60 percent is devoted to adult primary care, 30 percent to general pediatrics, and 10 percent to women's healthcare. Women's healthcare, for approximately 25 percent of family practitioners, is devoted to obstetrics (Lipsky 2003). However, the distribution of time can vary significantly in actual practice, depending on prevailing patterns and expectations in the region in question. In some markets, family practitioners devote a substantial portion of their practice to obstetrical care. In other markets, family practitioners provide no obstetrical care at all. The mix of family practitioners and general internists also varies widely from region to region, as illustrated in Table 3.1.

4. Failing to account for time physicians spend in activities other than patient care. Whether determining physician need or physician supply, the focus should be on time physicians spend on patient care activities (direct or indirect), not time spent on teaching, research, or administrative activities. Thus, physician-need ratios should be interpreted as the required number of physicians devoted full-time

Table 3.1. Number of Family Medicine and Internal Medicine Physicians Active in Patient Care in Selected Markets

Market	Family Medicine Physicians	Internal Medicine Physicians	Total Adult Primary Care Physicians	Family Medicine % of Total
Central CT, 2003	56	88	144	39
E. Central FL, 2004	102	86	188	54
Northern KY, 2003	131	37	168	78
W. Central NJ, 2002	46	111	157	29
Southern NJ, 2003	92	57	149	62
S. Central PA, 2003	293	66	359	82

Source: Health Strategies & Solutions, Inc. (Supply numbers assembled through various managed care and hospital web site directories.)

to patient care per 100,000 population. On the supply side, physicians who spend a substantial portion of time on teaching, research, or administration should be discounted or not counted at all, which makes it very difficult to apply physician-to-population ratios in an academic environment.

5. *Ignoring the effect of nonphysician clinicians.* The availability of nonphysician clinicians (NPCs), such as certified nurse practitioners or nurse midwives, varies substantially from region to region throughout the United States as shown in the Table 3.2.

Physician-to-population ratios should be adjusted downward in markets where the supply of NPCs is well above national norms in these categories. A convenient rule of thumb is that a full-time nonphysician clinician handles one-half to two-thirds the workload of a full-time-equivalent (FTE) physician. The upper end of the range is typical for practices where NPC use is relatively "mature," as evidenced by patient panels predominantly managed by the NPC or extensive delegation of clinical responsibility to the NPC.

6. *Ignoring the fact that many medical subspecialists devote some of their practice to primary care.* Some medical subspecialists spend 20 percent of their time providing primary care services to patients

Table 3.2. Nonphysician Clinician Supply per 100,000 Population by Region

	New England	South Atlantic	East North Central	West North Central	Pacific
Physician Assistants	14.0	10.2	7.8	16.7	8.1
Nurse Practictioners	48.5	23.8	17.9	38.5	24.6
Certified Nurse Midwives	4.2	2.1	1.8	2.8	1.7

Note: Physician assistant data are from 1999, nurse practitioner data are from 1998, and certified nurse midwife data are from 2000. Regions are as defined by the Bureau of Health Professions.

Source: U.S. Department of Health and Human Services, Bureau of Health Professions (2003).

under their care. From the standpoint of medical staff planning, such physicians should be counted as 0.2 general internists plus 0.8 FTEs in their respective subspecialties. Failing to make this adjustment often leads to overestimating both the shortage of general internists and the surplus of various medical subspecialties in a given market.

7. Not accounting for the role hospitalists play. Hospitalists are a rapidly growing specialty in many markets. In most cases, hospitalists function as internists, managing the entire inpatient stay of patients who would otherwise be cared for in the hospital by their community-based primary care physicians. In a few cases, hospitalists are subspecialists (usually in pulmonary medicine) who function as "intensivists," managing the care of all patients in the intensive care unit of a hospital. In either case, the contribution that hospitalists make toward meeting the community need for general internists or medical specialists should not be overlooked.

8. Inappropriately using a medical staff development plan to link investment in physician recruitment to additional referrals from physicians or to look at a hospital's strategic or economic needs rather than the community's needs. Regulatory agencies require that a hospital look at need from the perspective of a community, not from the hospital's strategic perspective. Thus a hospital may not have a sufficient number of subspecialists on its medical staff, but this does not necessarily translate to the broader community needing more subspecialists. Hospitals that ignore this requirement and offer recruitment incentives to physicians risk allegations of kickbacks and improper benefits under the tax laws (Glaser 2003).

The remainder of this chapter provides a guide to medical staff development planning and presents the range of factors that complicate attempts to quantify the current and future supply of physicians within a community or region or on a particular hospital medical staff.

OBJECTIVES OF MEDICAL STAFF DEVELOPMENT PLANNING

Medical staff development planning is a valuable tool for healthcare providers and serves the following purposes:

- *To complete the physician component of a community needs assessment.* In the past, designation as a health professional shortage area (HPSA) or medically underserved area (MUA) was a commonly accepted, objective means of demonstrating community need. Now, because the end product of a community needs assessment is an accounting of current and projected community-wide physician surpluses or deficits in as many as 25 or 30 different specialties, medical staff development plans provide a much more detailed profile of physician need tailored to a specific community.

   The first concern is whether enough physicians practice in the area to meet the current need within the communities served by the hospital. Sometimes, clear indicators of unmet need, such as long wait times for appointments with specialists or primary care practices closed to new patients, exist. However, boards of trustees also want to know that the number of physicians is sufficient to meet future community need. Future needs will be of particular concern if the area is experiencing rapid population growth, if several key members of the medical staff are approaching retirement age, or if the need for selected components of physician specialties (e.g., hand surgery within orthopedics) is unmet.

- *To define the size and composition of the medical staff organization.* Appropriate medical staff organization planning extends the community need analysis by accounting for the fact that individual hospitals and their medical staffs meet only a portion of the community's need. The key step is to adjust the population to be served to reflect the hospital's current or projected market share in each specialty. For example, if a hospital's market share is 60 percent in cardiology, the need for cardiologists on the hospital's medical staff arguably is only 60 percent of the community need for cardiologists.

- *To identify geographic-specific or subspecialty-specific physician needs.* A more detailed analysis can identify physician need in selected geographic subregions or selected physician subspecialties. Because geographic access to primary care physicians is an important consideration (i.e., patients have less tolerance for traveling long distances to access primary care physicians than for subspecialty care), the need for primary care physicians is often determined separately for the primary service area (PSA) and the secondary area (SSA) served by a hospital. Separately determining the need for medical (office-based) and interventional cardiologists (who spend most of their time in the cardiac catheterization laboratory) is an example of need determined at a subspecialty level.

- *To prioritize physician recruitment efforts.* Often, the most important outcome of a community or medical staff needs analysis is the identification of specialties where additional physicians need to be recruited to fill a current or projected deficit of one or more FTEs. Sometimes, the specialties assigned the highest recruitment priorities are those that have the largest numerical deficits. At other times, the highest priorities are assigned to specialties that are critical to growing market share in clinical programs that have the highest strategic importance to the hospital.

- *To identify specialties where competition for patients is likely to intensify because of projected physician surpluses.* In specialties with a projected physician surplus, further recruitment would only be warranted in special cases: when existing physicians are not achieving desired standards of quality or enabling access by patients in a timely manner; when a clinical program has very high strategic importance and the only way to capture market share from competitors is to recruit additional physicians in a related specialty; or when the unexpected retirement or departure of a key physician with a very busy practice creates an immediate need that cannot be met by the other physicians in the specialty.
- *To provide information to support physician growth plans.* Sophisticated and forward-thinking physician groups increasingly use medical staff planning methodologies to answer the following questions:
    —Should we add an associate to our practice? More specifically, will a new associate be able to build and maintain a viable patient base in light of the current and projected community need for physicians in our specialty?
    —Is the unmet need in communities within or contiguous to our primary market area sufficient to warrant opening a satellite office?
    —Is the population in the markets we serve (or desire to serve) sufficient to justify recruiting a subspecialist (e.g., an electrophysiologist, a surgical oncologist, or a hand surgeon)?

In summary, medical staff development plans may address physician need at multiple levels: the community at large; the hospital or health system medical staff; or individual physician practices.

Implementing the plan by filling needs identified during the medical staff planning process can benefit parties at all three levels. Having a well-developed plan in place also makes it easier to assist certain physician practices with recruitment and other practice support, assuming the plan has documented the underlying community need for additional physicians and has identified specialties where recruitment is a high priority.

A STEP-BY-STEP METHODOLOGY FOR DETERMINING PHYSICIAN NEED

In the simplest terms, medical staff planning consists of the following four steps:

1. Define the population to be served.
2. Determine the number of physicians required to meet the needs of that population at a specialty-specific level.
3. Compare the number of physicians needed with the available physician supply to identify and quantify surpluses and deficits specialty by specialty.
4. Decide which areas of shortage have the highest priority, and develop strategies to address these unmet needs.

As suggested at the beginning of this chapter, none of these steps is as simple as it sounds. In the remainder of the chapter, the four steps outlined above are expanded into a 17-step methodology for determining physician need at both the community and the hospital level. Approaches for addressing the many difficult issues that complicate the process are also discussed.

Before beginning the process of determining physician need, hospitals and health systems must address several key questions:

• Which set of the physician-to-population ratios is applicable to our market?

- How should the chosen set of ratios be adjusted to account for the unique characteristics of our region?
- What data can we use to develop a true understanding of the existing physician supply in the community?
- What do we know about how our own physicians practice? How many physicians work on a part-time basis? How many are close to retirement? How many patients do they refer to competitor hospitals? How much primary care is delivered by specialists? To what extent are nonphysician clinicians used?
- Who is responsible for determining which areas of need merit the highest priority? How should this be coordinated with other planning activities?

Step 1. Define the communities or geographic markets to be served. The communities or markets to be served may be a single county, multiple counties, a city, a metropolitan area, or any cluster of contiguous towns or zip codes that may fall within one or several geopolitical regions. To determine physician need for a hospital or health system, patient origin data can be used to subdivide the market into a PSA and one or more SSAs. Many hospitals define their PSA as the communities or zip codes where they derive the first 75 percent of their inpatient discharges, and the SSA(s) as the communities where the next 10 to 15 percent of their patients reside. While this approach may be suitable for some applications, it can lead to very misleading results when a program or specialty is truly regional in nature and draws a significantly higher percentage of patients from a much broader geographic area. An explanation of how to account for this situation is described later in this chapter.

2. Select a time horizon. The time horizon for medical staff development planning usually includes a baseline year and a forecast year. The baseline year is typically "next year"; the forecast year is usually three to five years later. This approach allows the plan to address both immediate and longer-term needs.

Step 3. Obtain current and projected population estimates. Current and projected population data should be obtained for each of the communities or geographic markets (or submarkets) identified in step 1. Because the age of the population being served is the single most important demographic factor affecting the utilization of physician services, population data should be obtained for the following four age groups: 0 to 14 years, 15 to 44, 45 to 64, and 65 and over. The description of step 5 illustrates how to adjust a set of baseline physician-to-population ratios to account for an unusual population age mix in a given market.

Step 4. Select a baseline set of physician-to-population ratios. As noted earlier, most of the recommended physician-to-population ratios that have appeared in the literature in recent years understate the need for medical and surgical specialists in most markets. Therefore, the current national distribution of physicians (MDs and DOs) by specialty and subspecialty, shown in Table 3.3, is a better point of departure. (Note that Table 3.3 does not include data for many specialties, including emergency medicine, anesthesiology, radiology, pathology, or psychiatry, but supply estimates can be found for these and other unlisted specialties from the same sources used to create Table 3.3.)

Using current physician supply ratios to define a baseline set of need ratios does not imply that supply and demand are in balance in all specialties at the national level. However, the current supply of physicians in a specialty (influenced as it is by market forces) is a better baseline measure of need than a physician-to-population ratio based on a model of how care *should* be delivered (e.g., GMENAC, COGME) or projections based on healthcare reform that never occurred.

The baseline set of ratios is only a point of departure. Several of the following steps suggest how to adjust the baseline ratios to reflect conditions in a given market. These adjustments are an essential element of the need methodology. No single set of ratios can be applied to all communities or all markets. Ratios that are appropriate in youthful, suburban Denver, Colorado, cannot be used in Arizona or Florida communities where 20 to 30 percent of the population is over the age of 65. Ratios that apply in Cleveland or Cincinnati,

Table 3.3. Physicians Active in Patient Care per 100,000 Population for Selected Specialties

Primary Care	
Family/General Practice	33.8
Internal Medicine	28.9
Pediatrics	14.9
Subtotal Primary Care	**77.7**
Medical Specialties	
Allergy/Immunology	1.2
Cardiology	6.5
Dermatology	3.1
Endocrinology	1.2
Gastroenterology	3.4
Hematology/Oncology	2.7
Infectious Disease	1.2
Nephrology	1.7
Neurology	3.4
Pulmonary Disease	2.5
Rheumatology	1.1
Subtotal Medical Specialties	**27.9**
Surgical Specialties	
Cardiovascular/Cardiothoracic	1.6
Colorectal Surgery	0.4
General Surgery	8.7
Hand Surgery	0.4
Neurosurgery	1.4
Obstetrics/Gynecology	12.6
Ophthalmology	5.9
Orthopedics	6.8
Otolaryngology	2.8
Plastic Surgery	2.0
Urology	3.1
Vascular Surgery	0.7
Subtotal Surgical Specialties	**46.6**

Source: Health Strategies & Solutions, Inc. Assembled from Pasko and Seidman (2003); U.S. Census Bureau (2004); Medical Marketing Service, Inc. (2003).

Ohio, should not be used in Akron or Dayton and are certainly not applicable in any of Ohio's 51 nonmetropolitan counties.

Step 5. Adjust baseline physician-to-population ratios to account for the age mix of the resident population. Table 3.4 shows the number of office visits per 100,000 population by age cohort to physicians in several medical and surgical disciplines.

Except for obstetrics/gynecology, office visit rates steadily increase as the population ages, but the ratio of the visit rate for persons age 65 and over compared to the visit rate for all ages varies significantly by specialty. In family medicine and orthopedics, for example, the office visit rate in the 65 and over age group is less than double the rate for all ages. But in internal medicine the ratio is more than 3 to 1, and in urology it is more than 4 to 1 (U.S. DHHS 2002).

If the age mix of the population in a given market closely mirrors the U.S. population, an adjustment of the baseline ratios for these or other specialties is unnecessary. However, if the percentage of residents age 65 and over is significantly higher or lower than the national average, the physician-to-population ratios should be adjusted accordingly.

Age-specific office visit rates derived from the data used to create Table 3.4 can be used to generate age-specific physician-to-population ratios. These results are shown for selected specialties in Table 3.5. In turn, age-specific physician ratios can be used to determine age-adjusted physician-to-population ratios for any community or region.

Step 6. Modify age-adjusted ratios to reflect unique characteristics of the local or regional marketplace. One characteristic that should be investigated in every market is the relative mix of physicians in family medicine, general practice, and internal medicine. Nationwide, according to the American Medical Association, 33 family and general practitioners per 100,000 persons were reported as of December 31, 2000, compared to 52 internists per 100,000 (35 general internists plus 17 in various subspecialties). In New England, however, internists outnumber family and general practitioners by 3 to

Table 3.4. Office Visits per 100,000 Population by Age Cohort for Selected Specialties

Specialty	0–14 Years	15–44 Years	45–64 Years	65+ Years	All Ages
Family Medicine	42,700	60,400	92,300	115,500	70,500
Internal Medicine	2,400	25,500	70,200	140,000	44,600
Gastroenterology	150	3,100	9,800	11,300	5,000
Neurology	450	1,900	4,400	6,700	2,800
Obstetrics/Gynecology	750	40,500	15,500	8,500	22,500
Orthopedic Surgery	7,000	14,300	21,500	26,400	15,900
Urology	850	2,300	8,800	28,400	6,600

Source: U.S. Department of Health and Human Services

1 (77 per 100,000 compared to 25). In the west north central states (Iowa, Kansas, Minnesota, Missouri, Nebraska, North Dakota, and South Dakota), on the other hand, family and general practitioners (43 per 100,000) outnumber internists (42 per 100,000) (Pasko and Seidman 2003).

Although family medicine physicians and internists are both typically classified as adult primary care physicians, they are not interchangeable, because the mix of patients they treat is very different. As noted earlier, the norm for family medicine physicians is to devote 60 percent of their practice to adult primary care, 30 percent to general pediatric care, and 10 percent to women's healthcare. The age-adjusted ratios for family medicine, general internal medicine, general pediatrics, and, in some cases, obstetrics should therefore be modified in markets with an atypical mix of family practitioners and internists.

Note that an altogether different set of ratios must be used in rural market areas, where the overall physician-to-population ratio is much lower, and the population base is usually too small to support even one physician in a number of medical and surgical specialties. Thus primary care physicians (family medicine, general

Table 3.5. Physicians Needed per 100,000 Population by Age for Selected Specialties

Specialty	0–14 Years	15–44 Years	45–64 Years	65+ Years
		29.0	44.3	
Family Medicine	20.5	16.5	45.5	55.4
Internal Medicine	1.5	2.1	6.6	90.7
Gastroenterology	0.1	2.4	5.4	7.7
Neurology	0.6	22.7	8.7	8.2
Obstetrics/Gynecology	0.4	6.2	9.3	4.8
Orthopedic Surgery	3.0	1.1	4.2	11.4
Urology	0.4			13.4

Source: U.S. Department of Health and Human Services (2002); Health Strategies & Solutions Inc. (2003).

practice, general internal medicine, and pediatrics) and physicians in more prevalent specialties (obstetrics, general surgery, and orthopedic surgery) account for a much higher proportion of the physician base in rural markets.

Ohio, for example, reported 23 family medicine and general practice physicians per 100,000 population in both metropolitan and nonmetropolitan areas. However, family medicine and general practice physicians accounted for only 9 percent of the physicians active in patient care in the metropolitan counties (23 out of 244 per 100,000), compared to 25 percent of the physicians active in patient care in the nonmetropolitan areas (23 out of 92 per 100,000) (Pasko and Seidman 2003).

Step 7. Multiply the current and projected community population by the appropriately adjusted physician-to-population ratios to determine communitywide physician need. The result of this straightforward analytical step is the number of physicians (active in patient care) required in each specialty to meet the current and future need in the community. For example, if six FTE cardiologists are needed per 100,000 population, a community with a population of

500,000 persons would require 30 FTE cardiologists active in patient care.

Step 8. Determine the supply of active physicians in the community, specialty by specialty. Numerous sources can be used to compile an inventory of physicians active in patient care in the community. These include hospital medical staff rosters, managed care physician panels (available on insurance company web sites), state licensure data, and state or regional medical society data. One must be careful using data from these sources, however. Directories are often out of date; specialties are often self-designated; and some physicians report multiple office locations or use home addresses instead of office addresses. Cross-checking information from the various data sources is strongly recommended.

Once a current inventory has been developed, an attempt should be made to project the future community supply of physicians in each specialty. The percentage of physicians age 60 and over (or age 55 and over) in a given specialty can be used to estimate retirements within the five-year planning horizon. New physicians who enter the market upon completing residency programs will add to the current supply. Established physicians who relocate to other markets or who retire from active practice at an early age (two phenomena accelerated by the current malpractice crisis in many states) will decrease the current supply.

Step 9. Calculate communitywide physician surpluses and deficits, specialty by specialty. This is a quantitative step. The current (projected) physician need in each specialty is subtracted from the current (projected) physician supply to determine current (projected) surpluses and deficits in each specialty.

Step 10. Reality test the results of the surplus/deficit analysis. In some cases, the results of step 9 for some specialties will be at odds with reality. Most often, this occurs when the quantitative need analysis indicates no need for additional physicians in a given specialty at the same time that other information clearly indicates a significant shortage. For example, the results of a community survey or focus group discussion carried out as part of a community health needs assessment may have indicated long wait times for appointments, many practices closed to new patients, or other service or coverage issues.

The first step in resolving such a situation is to verify that the estimated supply of physicians in the specialty is accurate. Confirm that all physicians in the inventory are still in active practice (full time or nearly full time) and that they have not relocated their practice to another community. Make necessary adjustments to the physician supply in the specialty, and recalculate the community-wide surplus or deficit. If the results are still inconsistent with demonstrated community need for additional physicians, further adjustments to the physician-to-population ratios may be warranted.

Step 11. Make a final determination of community need, and publish the results. Repeat steps 7, 8, and 9 to incorporate any changes in either physician supply or physician need that arise from step 10 (changes in need would result from any final adjustments to the physician-to-population ratios). Disseminate the community needs analysis (surpluses and deficits by specialty). Identify all data sources, provide the rationale for all calculations of physician supply, and specify all assumptions supporting the final set of physician-to-population ratios.

Step 12. Define the effective service population for each specialty represented on the hospital medical staff. No hospital or health system provides 100 percent of the medical care required by the residents of its PSA. Most hospitals have different market shares and different "out of area draw" in different specialties. Current market share and patient origin data can be used to calculate an effective service population for each specialty as shown in the examples below.

Suppose a hospital has a 40 percent market share in cardiology within its PSA, where the resident population is 500,000 people; and suppose that 20 percent of the hospital's cardiology patients live outside the PSA. This hospital would then have an "effective service population" of 250,000 persons in cardiology:

$$(500,000 * 0.4)/(1.0 - 0.2) = 250,000.$$

By way of comparison, if the same hospital has a 36 percent market share in pulmonary medicine and draws only 10 percent of its pulmonary patients from outside its PSA, its effective service population for pulmonary medicine would only be 200,000 persons:

$$(500,000 * 0.36)/(1.0 - 0.1) = 200,000$$

Step 13. Multiply the current and future effective service population for each specialty by the appropriate physician-to-population ratio for that specialty (as determined in steps 4, 5, 6, and 10) to determine physician need by specialty at the hospital level. This step is similar to step 7, except that the need in each specialty is determined by multiplying the appropriate physician-to-population ratio by the effective service population for the specialty instead of by the community-wide population. The result is the number of FTE physicians required in each specialty to meet the hospital's current and future need. Building on the example in step 12, if there is a need for 6 cardiologists per 100,000 population, a hospital with an effective service population of 250,000 in cardiology would require 15 FTE cardiologists.

Step 14. Determine the current supply of physicians on the hospital medical staff, specialty by specialty. This step is also more difficult than it seems. The starting point is to assemble a database for all physicians on the hospital's active medical staff. The database should identify each physician's age, specialty and practice group, as well as his or her activity at the hospital. Depending on the specialty, recent activity might include admissions (or discharges), number of inpatient and outpatient procedures performed, and total outpatient referrals.

The activity data are used to estimate each physician's current FTE contribution to the hospital. Activity levels can be compared across all physicians in a specialty or can be compared to published norms for each specialty. From the hospital's perspective, physicians should be counted as less than one FTE if their activity levels are well below expectations in a specialty. If physicians split their practice equally between two hospitals, for example, they should be counted as 0.5 FTE at each institution. Other physicians who fall into the partial FTE category are physicians who spend fewer hours in patient care than the average physician in their specialty, for any number of personal or lifestyle reasons. Conversely, a physician whose activity levels are far above norms for a specialty may be counted as contributing more than one FTE to the hospital.

Other adjustments should be made for medical subspecialists who are known to devote a significant proportion of their practice to primary care, or for surgeons who split their practice between two specialties (e.g., general surgery and vascular surgery). In this case, a physician's FTE contribution should be split between the appropriate specialties in proportion to the estimated time the physician devotes to each.

Step 15. Calculate surpluses or deficits on the hospital medical staff, specialty by specialty. This step is analogous to step 9, during which community-wide surpluses and deficits are determined. The current (projected) physician need in each specialty (from step 13) is subtracted from the current (projected) physician supply (from step 14) to determine current (projected) surpluses and deficits by specialty on the hospital medical staff.

Step 16. Reality test the results of the surplus/deficit analysis. As in the community needs analysis, the results of step 15 for a few specialties might seem at odds with reality, most often when the quantitative need analysis indicates no need for additional physicians in a given specialty at the same time that other information clearly indicates a shortage. In this case, the information at hand will be more specific to the practices represented on the hospital medical staff. For example, primary care physicians may have identified several specialties where there are long wait times for routine consultations; or, one or more busy practices in a particular specialty may be in search of new associates.

Usually, the key to resolving such situations is to verify that the estimated supply of physicians in each specialty is accurate. Confirm that the original estimate of each physician's FTE contribution (based on activity levels and assumed loyalty to the hospital) accurately reflects the way physicians on the medical staff are practicing. Also, confirm that the specialty assignments are accurate, especially in the case of physicians who have been assigned partial FTE designation in two different specialties.

Step 17. Make a final determination of physician surpluses and deficits by specialty at the hospital level and publish the results. After making any necessary adjustments to the physician supply, recalculate the current and projected physician surplus or deficit in each specialty for the hospital medical staff. This final set of surpluses and deficits defines the need for current and future additions to the medical staff.

IMPLEMENTATION STRATEGIES

Often, a medical staff development plan is accompanied by a series of implementation strategies designed to ensure that identified needs are met in timely fashion. Many implementation strategies focus on recruitment and retention of physicians in specialties where strategic priorities are highest or quantitative needs are greatest.

Recruitment Strategies

A thorough medical staff development plan can provide rationale to demonstrate that specialty needs are unmet, or will likely be unmet, as a result of physician retirement, population growth, or socioeconomic changes, and that recruitment, therefore, is justified. Example approaches to recruitment include the following strategies.

Reimburse recruitment, relocation, and practice start-up expenses
The Internal Revenue Service permits hospitals to pay reasonable recruitment and relocation expenses as long as an independent, objective determination of community need has been conducted and documented (e.g., by using a thorough medical staff development

planning process). The actual recruitment, relocation, and practice start-up expenses must be reasonable, given the physician specialty and the applicable market, and structured appropriately. These arrangements are only applicable to physicians who are recruited to provide incremental supply to meet current or projected community need, meaning that practices that are currently in a service area are ineligible.

Physicians who relocate their practices to a new community or physicians who are finishing training (e.g., residents and fellows) are eligible. "Allowable and standard" recruitment and relocation expenses may include expenses incurred for house hunting, for temporary housing while actively locating permanent housing, for realtor commissions, for closing costs, for travel for house hunting, and during a transition period of relocation. In some cases, income support, structured as advances to loans (see below) is a component of recruitment and relocation packages. These arrangements are actually loans used to provide salary guarantees and, if properly structured, may meet the conditions and requirements of reasonable payments (Glaser 2003).

As with any payment for recruitment, all payments need to be documented as reasonable and not be construed in any manner to improperly induce referrals to the payer of the expenses (i.e., a hospital or health system). For more information on relocation and recruitment expense payments, legal counsel should be consulted, particularly since laws and regulations change almost daily (Glaser 2003).

Use local recruitment and headhunter firms whenever possible
Local firms have a far superior advantage in touting to a candidate the benefits of moving to a particular area, based on local knowledge about schools, housing areas, and other lifestyle considerations.

Offer real estate down payments as part of recruitment packages
These down payments are a component of a total compensation package and can be structured as an advance on a loan or salary guarantee.

Whenever possible, recruit to established practices that are loyal to the hospital

Recruiting to loyal practices will increase the likelihood that the new recruit will be the beneficiary of mentoring and be loyal to the hospital sponsoring the recruitment assistance. These arrangements must be structured with extreme care given the potential for benefit to flow to the existing practices (and not just to the recruited physicians). Legal counsel should be consulted prior to entering into these types of arrangements.

Offer malpractice expense relief

Offering malpractice insurance relief should be a key consideration when your state is designated as a malpractice crisis state. Several alternatives can be considered in this approach. Again, legal counsel should provide specific advice.

Recruit to practices that are "ancillary rich"

Ancillary-rich practices will have the resources to offer attractive compensation to recruits.

Recruit to practices where demonstrated community need from the physician need analysis is highest

Strategically recruiting to such practices will reduce the time required for the new physician to achieve financial viability.

Retention strategies are described in detail in Chapter 5, which addresses a wide array of ways a hospital or health system can earn the loyalty of private practice physicians.

The medical staff development planning process can be used (or abused) to suit any number of agendas. But when the appropriate analyses and methodical approaches, such as the ones described in this chapter, are followed, hospitals, physicians, and patients should all benefit by having a physician population that is tailored to better meet community needs.

REFERENCES

Cooper, R. A. 2002. "There's a Shortage of Specialists. Is Anyone Listening?" *Academic Medicine* 77 (8): 761–66.

———. 1995. "Perspectives on the Physician Workforce to the Year 2020." *Journal of the American Medical Association* 274 (19): 1534–43.

Cooper, R. A., T. E. Getzen, H. J. McKee, and P. Laud. 2002. "Economic and Demographic Trends Signal an Impending Physician Shortage." *Health Affairs* 21 (1): 140–54.

Council on Graduate Medical Education. 2003a. "Minutes of Meeting, September 17, 2003." [Online article; retrieved 11/19/2003.] http://www.cogme.gov /minutes09_03.htm.

———. 2003b. "Minutes of Meeting, April 10–11, 2003." [Online article; retrieved 11/19/2003.] http://www.cogme.gov/minutes04_03.htm.

———. 1999. "Summary of Fourteenth Report: COGME Physician Workforce Policies: Recent Developments and Remaining Challenges in Meeting National Goals." [Online article; retrieved 5/28/1999.] http://www.cogme.gov/rpt14.htm.

———. 1996. "Summary of Eighth Report: Patient Care Physician Supply and Requirements: Testing COGME Recommendations." [Online article; retrieved 5/28/1999.] http://www.cogme.gov/rpt8.htm.

———. 1995. "Summary of Sixth Report: Managed Health Care: Implications for the Physician Workforce and Medical Education." [Online article; retrieved 5/28/1999.] http://www.cogme.gov/rpt6.htm.

———. 1992. "Summary of Third Report: Improving Access to Health Care Through Physician Workforce Reform: Directions for the 21st Century." [Online article; retrieved 11/19/2003.] http://www.cogme.gov/rpt3.htm.

Glaser, L. 2003. Personal interview, December 12.

Graduate Medical Education National Advisory Committee. 1980. *Report of the Graduate Medical Education National Advisory Committee to the Secretary, U.S. Department of Health and Human Services*, vol. 1. Washington, DC: Office of Graduate Medical Education, U.S. DHHS.

Health Strategies & Solutions, Inc. 2003. Company databases.

Kronick, R., D. C. Goodman, J. Wennberg, and E. Wagner. 1993. "The Marketplace in Health Care Reform: The Demographic Limitations of Managed Competition." *New England Journal of Medicine* 328 (2): 148–52.

Lipsky, M. 2003. Personal interview, November 3.

Medical Marketing Service, Inc. 2003. Database of American Osteopathic Association Nonfederal Physicians in Patient Care.

Pasko, T., and B. Seidman. 2003. *Physician Characteristics and Distribution in the United States, 2002–2003 Edition.* Chicago: American Medical Association.

Rivo, M. L., and D. A. Kindig. 1996. "A Report Card on the Physician Work Force in the United States." *New England Journal of Medicine* 334 (14): 892–96.

Schroeder, S. A. 1996. "How Can We Tell Whether There Are Too Many or Too Few Physicians? The Case for Benchmarking." *Journal of the American Medical Association* 276 (22): 1841–43.

U.S. Census Bureau. 2004. "State and County *QuickFacts.* [online article; retrieved 1/14/2004.] http://quickfacts.census.gov/gfd/staes/00000.html.

U.S. Department of Health and Human Services. 2002. "2000 National Ambulatory Medical Care Survey." CD-ROM Series 13, Number 32.

U.S. Department of Health and Human Services, Bureau of Health Professions. 2003. "State Health Workforce Profiles." [Online article; posted 12/2000; retrieved 12/2/03.] http://bhpr.hrsa.gov/healthworkforce/reports/profiles/.

Weiner, J. P. 1994. "Forecasting the Effects of Health Reform on US Physician Workforce Requirement." *Journal of the American Medical Association* 272 (3): 222–30.

CHAPTER 4

Creating Incentives for Participation in Medical Staff Organizations

In the past, when contribution margins for practice activities were higher, physicians were more willing to invest time in hospital-related activities. Today, however, with the increased availability of other care settings and the need to maximize revenue generation, physicians may be reluctant to sacrifice office time with their patients to attend to hospital matters.

—*Health Care Advisory Board (1999)*

AS PHYSICIANS HAVE to work increasingly long hours to achieve stable or declining practice revenue, how can hospitals and systems create incentives for physicians to actively participate in medical staff organizations? The solutions are not quick and easy, and a one-size-fits-all approach is inappropriate. Hospitals and systems will need to dig deep to find creative and perhaps unique incentives so that loosely aligned or independent physicians are motivated to participate actively in medical staff organizations. If healthcare organizations fail to create these incentives, the trends and influences discussed in Chapter 2 will likely lead to further separatism and alienation of physicians from hospitals and systems, and less participation, formally or informally, in medical staff functions and initiatives.

Less substantive participation on a medical staff means fewer physician candidates to serve as leaders or champions for critical functions of the medical staff and less involvement in service line planning, growth and development, and quality initiatives across the continuum of care.

Disenfranchised physicians are more likely to strip ancillary services from hospitals, leading to acrimonious and even hostile physician-hospital relationships. A lack of participation on the medical staff can also fuel a decline in referral relationships to a hospital and its affiliated physicians and, ultimately, diminished financial viability of a hospital or system.

Hospitals and health systems cannot sit idly by and let their medical staff organizations dwindle into irrelevancy. Examples abound of the deleterious effects of being passive and reacting to initiatives as they occur. Healthcare organizations instead must be proactive in revitalizing their medical staff organizations. This chapter will examine ways that hospitals and systems can create incentives for participation rather than continuing to passively observe the separation of physicians from traditional medical staff organizations.

LAYING THE GROUNDWORK FOR INCENTIVES

Numerous incentives are available for hospitals and systems to motivate physician participation in the programs, services, and initiatives of medical staff organizations. These incentives should motivate physicians to be truly active participants in the medical staff organizations, not inactive, marginally active, passive, or ambivalent participants, or worse yet, combatants with a hospital in a competitive relationship.

Whether or not these incentives will be effective is largely dependent on the climate and environment in which the physician-hospital relationship operates. The success of incentives is primarily a function of the level of trust already created and perceived, the actual value-added benefits from past participation on the medical staff, and earlier successful initiatives of the medical staff (e.g., attainment of quality metrics). Further, if a healthcare organization has achieved organization-wide market leverage, the hospital or system is also able to have more leverage with aligned physicians and is capable of offering more incentives.

A fundamental platform of trust and mutual benefit and an environment conducive to offering incentives for participation in the medical staff organization must exist before the incentives are rolled out. Otherwise, offering incentives may be a waste of time and resources. Incentives are also likely to be more effective in combinations of two or more; the likelihood that offering only one carrot will lead to increased participation of physicians in the medical staff is slim.

PHYSICIAN LOYALTY AND INCENTIVES

An incentive, by definition, is something that moves people to action. Voluminous amounts of research have been conducted on what motivates human behavior. Of note are several studies conducted specifically on what fosters physician loyalty. Loyalty may not necessarily translate into motivation for active physician involvement in a medical staff organization, but it is a good starting point for examining physician perspectives on why they choose to be loyal to one hospital and system over another, and how incentives to gain significant involvement in the medical staff organization might be structured based on these drivers of loyalty.

The Health Care Advisory Board conducted two studies that evaluate the drivers of physician loyalty. The first study was an 86-question survey sent to 2,663 specialists in nine specialties; 530 responses to the survey were received, for a response rate of 20 percent. The survey reported that the rankings of key drivers of physician loyalty to hospital were reported to be the following (Holder and Cochran 2003):

1. Expertise of other physicians on staff
2. Nursing competence
3. Hospital efficiency
4. Hospital reputation and financial condition
5. Clinical practice support
6. Commitment to innovative technology
7. Hospital administration and decision making
8. Income considerations

In another report by the Health Care Advisory Board, entitled *The Physician Perspective—Understanding the Basis of Physician Facility Selection (and Defection)*, physicians were asked to rate the importance of various major factors to determine hospital facility selection. The findings indicated that the two key drivers for physician loyalty are proximity to office and competence of nursing staff, followed closely by the reputation (a variation of the expertise factor cited in Holder and Cochran [2003]) of physicians (Health Care Advisory Board 1999).

Messinger and Welter (2003) suggest the following five drivers of physician loyalty:

1. Superior hospital customer service and quality
2. A culture that supports medical staff participation in decision making and planning
3. Technologies that are of practical use to physicians
4. Meaningful physician practice support
5. Ongoing referral tracking and management

The common theme is that hospitals and systems that maintain efficient operations and systems and high-quality nursing staffs, and as a result attract high-quality physicians, are well-positioned to create an array of incentives that will encourage strong physician alignment to a medical staff. In a sense, hospitals with these characteristics become magnets for physicians.

16 INCENTIVES FOR ACTIVE PARTICIPATION IN THE MEDICAL STAFF ORGANIZATION

What incentives will motivate physicians to move beyond affiliation or loyalty to energetic participation in program growth and development, active clinical referral relationships, and deep commitment to hospital or system strategic initiatives?

The remainder of this chapter describes many examples of incentives for medical staff organization participation, including strategies for initiating participation and encouraging more extensive or more active participation in the medical staff organization. As with any physician strategy employed by a hospital or system, the specific incentives selected must take into consideration past successes, current capabilities, existing benefits for physicians and the sponsoring hospital or system, and the likelihood of future success. In some cases, the collateral damage that may ensue if certain incentives are offered and fail is often worse than not having offered the incentives at all.

1. Provide access to efficient operations and systems. One of the most prevalent reasons physicians develop ambulatory surgery centers, independent hospitals, and other out-of-hospital services is to create more efficient operations and systems designed to meet their special needs. Operations and systems efficiency is a necessity, not an option, for hospital management. Examples of operations efficiency include effectiveness of imaging scheduling, emergency room wait times, operating room turnaround time, efficacy of cardiac diagnostic tests, turnaround time for lab results (can the hospital match the commercial lab standard of same-day results reporting?), and efficient scheduling and results reporting of other diagnostic and treatment services.

The watchword here is *efficiency*. The physician community is troubled by inefficient and expensive hospital consumption of resources. According to Stuart Brogadir, M.D., "It is important to change the size, scope, and resource consumption of hospitals. Physicians have had to make major changes in practice patterns due to a constrained reimbursement environment, coupled with escalating practice expenses. Physicians will only have interest and trust in a potential hospital partner that is able to demonstrate efficient operations and systems, not expensive and wasteful staffing and infrastructure" (Brogadir 2003).

2. Promote and communicate a vision. A hospital or system should promote a compelling vision for the future and establish a reasonable and realistic time frame, such as three to five years, to achieve the vision. The vision statement and the associated activities needed to achieve the vision must be seen as a tangible commitment to building an organization that truly values its physicians, otherwise these efforts will be seen as smoke and mirrors. According to Richard Afable, M.D., "Without a compelling vision, this may appear to be marketing tactics and techniques" (Afable 2003). Hospitals and systems should consider fostering a preferred position for participating physicians as the vision is rolled out.

3. Offer preferred malpractice coverage. Some fortunate hospitals with adequate financial reserves are able to offer preferred malpractice coverage or rates to physicians who participate on their medical staff. The difference in coverage or premium levels can be substantial. For example, Stamford Hospital in Stamford, Connecticut, has a formal affiliation with New York–Presbyterian Hospital, a tertiary academic medical center located in New York City. Through its affiliation with New York–Presbyterian Hospital, Stamford Hospital is able to access better malpractice coverage for physicians affiliated with Stamford. Stamford Hospital requires that physicians on its medical staff have the coverage of an A-rated insurance company, according to David Smith, senior vice president for strategy and market development at Stamford. According to Smith (2003), "About 200 of our physicians belonged to an insurance carrier that was downgraded to a B rating. Through an affiliation with New York–Presbyterian Hospital, they were able to make their captive available to physicians on our staff. It is not necessarily cheaper, and the physicians must qualify for coverage, but it is A rated."

Malpractice crisis states and specialties most affected by skyrocketing insurance costs provide a particular opportunity for hospitals to provide physician malpractice coverage relief.

4. Provide access to hospitalist programs and services. Another incentive to participate actively in the medical staff organization rather than remain independent is access to a hospitalist program. The use of hospitalists and hospitalist programs is on the rise. *Health News Digest* reports the number of hospitalists in 2003 to be more than 7,000 and predicts that almost 20,000 hospitalists will be in practice by 2010 (*Health News Digest* 2003).

Hospitalists are practicing at virtually all of the country's leading hospitals including Beth Israel Medical Center in New York City; Brigham and Womens Hospital in Boston; Cedars-Sinai Medical Center in Los Angeles; the Cleveland Clinic; Columbia-Presbyterian Medical Center in New York City; Emory University Hospital in Atlanta; the Mayo Clinic in Rochester, Minnesota; University of California San Francisco Medical Center; University of Chicago Hospitals; University of Iowa in Iowa City; University of Michigan Health System in Ann Arbor; and University of Pennsylvania Health System in Philadelphia.

In published studies, the average reduction in hospital costs and length of stay was about 15 percent (Wachter and Goldman 2002). Initially physicians are often reluctant to relinquish the inpatient component of patient care and associated revenue, but according to data from the American Academy of Family Physicians, by 2001, approximately 20 percent of its members were using hospitalists (Jackson 2001).

Primary care physicians are discovering that coming to the hospital each day to conduct rounds on only a few patients can be an inefficient use of time and a financial drain. According to Robert Wachter, M.D., president of the National Association of Inpatient Physicians and the person who coined the term *hospitalist* in a 1996 *New England Journal of Medicine* article, physicians' growing acceptance of hospitalists comes in part from the economic advantages the specialty offers. Wachter cited research showing that physicians who refer their inpatients to hospitalists can see their incomes rise between $20,000 and $47,000 annually (Maguire 2001).

Hospitalists offer physicians a range of benefits, from the ability to transfer call coverage responsibility to emergency and hospitalist physicians, to the ability to focus on one aspect of clinical practice. Health First, a multihospital system in Melbourne, Florida, instituted a hospitalist program at its flagship hospital, Holmes Regional Medical Center. According to Roy Wright, chief executive officer for the affiliated Cape Canaveral Hospital, "like other hospitalist programs, use of the hospitalist program at Holmes is strictly voluntary. The intention is to provide better patient management, and to eliminate one of the burdens of private practice—inpatient coverage" (Wright 2003).

5. Obtain an advanced information system. Hospital and health system attempts at physician practice management were largely failures, but they did demonstrate a valued capability: assisting physicians in improving practice efficiency and reducing costs through the use of information technology.

The evolution of information systems in hospitals and health systems is rapid and dramatic. Since 2000, hospitals have increased their reliance on information systems for patient preregistration, prescription renewal, and appointment scheduling. For physicians and nurses, information system advancements have grown considerably in areas of patient information access (e.g., medical records, medical histories, nurses' notes, patient demographics), test order entry, and test result viewings (Solovy 2002).

Many hospitals have, or are contemplating, implementation of electronic medical records (EMRs). A recent survey of physician practices by the Medical Group Management Association and Pfizer Health Solutions found that implementation of an EMR system resulted in an increase in payment levels of 26 percent, an increase in patient volume of 21 percent, and an improvement in patient and provider satisfaction scores of 31 percent and 50 percent, respectively (Messinger and Welter 2003). Almost all new hospital construction incorporates electronic order entry in the facility design components of information systems. With such potential to benefit both hospitals and physicians, could any incentive for active physician involvement in medical staff organizations be more motivating than advanced information systems, particularly an EMR system?

Key advantages of EMR include physician access to patient records from multiple locations; this improves overall access and makes the access more seamless by providing reports and results in near real time. In particular, physicians are demanding web-based access to laboratory and diagnostic information, meaning physician access anywhere, anytime.

Physicians who are preferred partners of the Covenant Health System in Milwaukee, Wisconsin, have access to an information system, which includes an EMR. This EMR enables access to core patient data (not the entire medical record) including a patient problem list, specialists seen, emergency room problem list, medications, and other variables.

Electronic order entry has been touted as a contributor to higher quality and more efficient care. A study by the California HealthCare Foundation and First Consulting Group compiled information from ten community hospitals that have made significant progress in automating their order entry process. According to this study "the carrot works better than the stick for community hospitals to go from the notepad to the computer" since community hospitals have looser relationships with affiliated physicians than do academic medical centers. In other words, physicians need to be convinced that electronic order entry will add value and efficiency to their practice (Benko 2003).

Community hospitals generally do not have the clout to attempt what Cedars-Sinai Medical Center in Los Angeles did early in 2003. Cedars-Sinai attempted to require that all of its 1,800 physicians use its new multimillion-dollar order entry system. Those who did not faced suspension of medical staff privileges. After an overwhelming number of complaints, this requirement was abandoned, for the time being (Benko 2003).

Physicians at the Via Christi Regional Medical Center in Wichita, Kansas, can access digital images, lab results, and clinical documentation on the Internet through a remote access system purchased by the medical center (*Health Management Technology* 2003). Physicians at Reid Hospital, a 240-bed not-for-profit located in Indiana, can access patient listings, vital signs, clinical progress notes, patient histories, physical examinations, prior admission data, laboratory results, and diagnostic radiology interpretation reports through the Internet using a security token (Kinyon 2003).

Another innovative concept was enacted by Strong Memorial Hospital in Rochester, New York. Strong offers affiliated physicians access to continuing education through its web site. Any member of the active medical staff of Strong or its affiliated hospitals is able to access continuing education material through its web site—day, evening, or night.

High cost is one of the key obstacles hospitals and systems face as they pursue state-of-the-art information systems that link various components of a healthcare system with affiliated physician practices. Both the initial capital and ongoing operating costs can be substantial. For example, the costs of implementing an electronic order entry system can be as high as $8 million for a 500-bed hospital that does not need major network upgrades. Annual maintenance can average $1.4 million (Kuperman and Gibson 2003).

6. Provide high-quality, measurable inpatient hospital care. Increasingly, hospitals and healthcare systems are coveting the various designations of high-quality status, such as those touted on HealthGrades.com or published in *U.S. News & World Report.* However, while the healthcare community may perceive that patients prefer to be cared for by high-quality hospitals and physicians, patients themselves may not feel so strongly. In other words, the public may not generally accept or appreciate the importance of being designated a high-quality provider. According to the Leapfrog Group, a coalition of large employers that is one of the leaders in the measurable pursuit of quality by healthcare providers, "We have a long way to go before we know consumers will use [the quality rankings]." According to a Harris poll conducted in October 2002, 25 percent of respondents said they had seen hospital ranking reports, but only 3 percent used them in making decisions about which facility to use (Fong 2003).

These quality ratings are, however, meaningful to healthcare providers. Providers are seeing more of their pay tied to performance based on quality measures and other contractual objectives (Fong 2003). More and more, payers and purchasers are working together to tie provider compensation to performance. For example, in 2002, Empire Blue Cross and Blue Shield in New York, and four of its largest clients—IBM, Pepsico, Verizon, and Xerox—paid a total of $195,000 to 29 hospitals that met at least one of two patient safety standards promoted by the Washington, DC–based Leapfrog Group. The standards to be met were implementation of a computerized order entry system and use of board-certified specialists in intensive care units (Fong 2003). According to Steven Safyer, M.D., chief medical officer of Montefiore Medical Center in the Bronx, New York, "We certainly didn't invest in a $100 million system for $50,000. We did it because it was the right thing to do" (Fong 2003).

The Virtua Health System in New Jersey has negotiated premium payments from its most prevalent HMO payer for achievement of three quality results. The sum total of bonus payments can be 3 percent of total HMO payments. Medicare is also planning to award bonuses to hospitals for providing superior care (McGinley 2003). Hospitals will submit data on patients with eight medical conditions, including stroke, heart attack, hip surgery, pneumonia, and heart failure. Hospitals that achieve top scores on quality would get small bonuses (e.g., 1 or 2 percent) in addition to regular Medicare payments. In the words of Thomas Scully, former head of the Centers for Medicare & Medicaid Services, "there's no question that pay for performance will work" (McGinley 2003).

Pay for performance could have key implications for physicians who choose to remain employed by a hospital or aligned to a medical staff organization. Employed physicians could be eligible for additional bonus pay as a result of achieving quality standards. Independent, aligned physicians, while not eligible for bonus pay, could ultimately benefit because the hospital would have more financial wherewithal to invest in other programs and services that benefit individual, independent physicians. The White House Office of Management and Budget is taking a harsher approach, suggesting financial penalties for hospitals and systems that demonstrate poor performance on quality measures.

7. Create a high-quality nursing program. As discussed earlier in this chapter, high-quality nursing staff and coverage are key drivers for physician loyalty. Hospitals and systems dedicated to creating active, committed medical staff organizations must ensure that they have a stable cadre of highly qualified nurses and also make wise choices about the trade-offs of having nurses care for a higher volume of patients. Are the cost savings generated from having fewer nurses on units significant enough to compromise patient care and physician satisfaction?

Stamford Hospital recently announced a program to move to a 4 to 1 nurse staffing ratio (i.e., four patients for every floor nurse), assigning significantly fewer patients per nurse than seen in other parts of the country. A 6 to 1 standard was enacted in July 2002 in California. The California Nurses Association lobbied for a 3 to 1 ratio, while the California Healthcare Association argued for a 10 to 1 ratio on medical/surgical units; the enacted 6 to 1 level was a compromise position supported by former California governor Gray Davis (Coile 2003).

The Main Line Health System in suburban Philadelphia also has boosted its efforts to retain nurses with the theory that a stable cadre of nursing staff will lead to higher quality of coverage. Nurses who stay with the system for a three-year period, in any of four hospitals, are eligible for a $25,000 retention bonus, payable in annual increments of $3,000, $7,000, and $15,000.

8. Make the medical staff bylaws residency requirement more lenient. One of the "disincentives" that medical staff organizations have historically instituted is restrictive residency requirements for membership on a medical staff. For example, Hunterdon Medical Center in Flemington, New Jersey, historically restricted its active medical staff privileges exclusively to physicians whose full-time office practices were within the same county as the hospital; this policy is now under review.

Hospitals may also restrict membership by instituting travel time limits. For example, a hospital may require a physician to reside within a certain number of minutes of a facility or within a defined distance from a hospital to ensure that calls will be covered on a timely basis. Exempla Lutheran Medical Center and Exempla Saint Joseph Hospital, both in the Denver, Colorado, metropolitan area, require a physician to be accessible for on-call coverage, which is defined as being within a 30-minute drive of the hospital where the physician is on call.

Many physicians perceive any standards (other than on-call distance and time requirements) to be too stringent and consider such requirements a disincentive for recruitment. As a result, many hospitals are revising residency requirements to eliminate this disincentive for medical staff membership. Stamford Hospital limited membership on its active medical staff to those physicians located in the hospital's primary service area, but it is considering ways to liberalize the physician residency requirements to eliminate a substantial disincentive for medical staff membership. The reconsideration will extend the opportunity for medical staff membership to a broader range of physicians. Otherwise, according to David Smith (2003), the policy "limits Stamford Hospital's ability to develop programs and services targeted to other zip codes that comprise a secondary and extended service area."

9. Provide access to recruitment and retention assistance. Hospitals often offer physician recruitment and retention programs and services, particularly when supported by an objective community needs assessment (for formal "health professional shortage area" and "medically underserved area" designation) as discussed in Chapter 3 of this book. Programs typically include a salary guarantee or subsidy, structured as a loan to a practice, which is forgiven if the physician remains in the underserved community providing service for a defined period.

These programs and benefits are typically only available to physicians with active medical staff status. According to Lou Glaser, Esq., "Care must be exercised in structuring recruitment arrangements. The goal is to provide the community with a needed service, and to not benefit existing physicians in an area of competitive advantage for a hospital but for which there is not community need" (Glaser 2003).

10. Provide access to practice transition and mentor stipends. William Beaumont Hospital in suburban Detroit, Michigan, offers a unique program to provide an incentive for an established, community-based physician to mentor a junior, start-up physician (usually a graduate of a residency program) and receive additional income for taking on this task. For a modest annual stipend of $20,000 to $30,000, the mentor physician trains a junior physician in clinical practice methods, staff supervision, and other practice management concepts. Eligibility for these mentor stipends historically has only been for physicians in areas and specialties deemed appropriate for the program and for active medical staff members of the hospital.

11. Offer access to the halo effect. Physicians are well aware that affiliation with high-quality, branded healthcare organizations can enhance their standing within the healthcare community. The halo effect of aligning with the "must have" hospital can also translate to higher patient volumes. Providers such as the Mayo Clinic and Cleveland Clinic have reputations for high-quality care that enable them to attract patients from around the world. Managed care plans are compelled to include these providers on their provider panels to meet purchaser demand, an advantage that provides financial benefits to physicians associated with these organizations by providing access to a significantly larger patient base (Rovinsky 2002).

12. Provide preferential access to the operating room. Some hospitals require active medical staff status to access any operating room time on the schedule; however, more inclusive scheduling or providing the most desirable time (e.g., early morning times on Monday through Friday) and staff (e.g., anesthesia, nursing) is often granted to the most active medical staff physicians.

13. *Offer advertising and promotion for preferred physicians.* Physicians actively aligned with a medical staff organization should also benefit from participation in hospital-sponsored practice promotion and advertising. Often, physician practices equate advertising and promotion as exposure in the yellow pages, on television and radio, and on billboards. However, Demby (1991) suggests that a more personal, high-touch presence such as arranging for physician speeches to community groups and other methods that establish a personal connection to patients, allowing physicians to meet and become acquainted with physician colleagues, and tailoring direct-mail pieces to promote the practice may be more effective than newspaper and yellow pages advertising.

Other techniques include the promotion of a hospital and its affiliated physicians to realtors and personnel departments of area employers, each of whom have access to new families moving to an area. Hospital web sites with "find a physician" links are also becoming common. At the Lovelace Health System located in Albuquerque, New Mexico, healthcare consumers can query the hospital's online database of medical staff physicians and search by specialty and physician location. Memorial Hospital in Gulfport, Mississippi, takes the search process a step further by allowing consumers to search by physician name and distance from a particular location like a home or business address.

14. *Facilitate strong and preferred referral relationships.* Although referral relationships are mostly built around clinical lines, many hospitals and systems recommend that primary care physicians who are employed by or have other integrated relationships with the hospital refer patients to specialists who are also aligned, rather than competitive, with the hospital. According to Leo Brideau, FACHE, chief executive officer of the Columbia St. Mary's Health System in Milwaukee, Wisconsin, "This is one of the most powerful potential

'carrots' if done effectively" (Brideau 2003). However, encouraging such referrals can be a challenge. Often, primary care physicians and specialists do not maintain strong professional relationships and do not know each others' capabilities. Specialists do not know what primary care physicians are looking for and why they might refer to a specialist affiliated with another hospital. Hospitals that facilitate face-to-face professional interaction between primary care physicians and specialists can usually make substantial inroads with this issue.

There are legal considerations when employing this approach. According to Lou Glaser, Esq., "This concept is about fostering relationships rather than forcing these relationships through direct economic incentives, which in turn raises legal issues. The concept is appropriate if it is all about service and easing practice for physicians" (Glaser 2003).

15. Provide access to supplemental income. Access to supplemental income can be offered to physicians by the hospital as a portion of technical revenue through joint ventures or other economic models, such as medical directorships and medical services agreements. Physicians who are active participants of medical staff organizations should be first in line for consideration of potential formal business relationships with the sponsoring hospital or system. These formal business relationships can be of economic value to the physicians who participate, to the extent that the declines in compensation can be offset by additional income generated by these formal business relationships.

According to Stuart Brogadir, M.D. (2003), "One of the best methods of aligning the interests of a hospital and its physicians is to truly partner in the provision of ambulatory care services."

Technical or ancillary revenue can, in some cases, represent 15 to 20 percent of total practice revenue. For ancillary service–rich practices (e.g., oncology, radiology, and gastroenterology), ancillary revenue can represent 30 to 35 percent or more of total practice income.

Historically, many of these ancillary procedures, and their associated technical revenue, were coveted and protected by hospital leaders. Yet in many instances the provision of ambulatory services out of the traditional hospital setting can be considered inevitable. By developing business relationships with physicians, and ultimately sharing the associated ancillary revenue, hospitals can use the resulting goodwill to offset the potential loss of other referral relationships for inpatient and outpatient services in the same or related service lines. Overall, it is far better to partner in the provision of those services that will inevitably migrate than drawing a line in the sand and naively believing that services can be retained in a hospital.

The array of economic business relationships can include economic joint ventures, lease arrangements, medical services agreements, or payment for time associated with program or service development. A strong incentive for physicians to participate in medical staff organizations is created when physicians are required to be on the active medical staff in order to be eligible for consideration as potential business partners. Again these types of relationships raise key legal considerations. Lou Glaser, Esq., notes that "It is important to distinguish between tying participation in a venture to referrals or business in general and doing business with those who buy into your philosophy. Limiting participation to those who will generate referrals or business raises significant legal issues. Nonetheless, hospitals can select as potential business partners those physicians who share the hospital's goals and objectives for the venture, for patient care, and for the community" (Glaser 2003).

16. Enable access to premium reimbursement rates. If the physician community, through a hospital-aligned independent practice association (IPA) or similar structure, can effectively negotiate with payers, then the physician community can often secure favorable reimbursement levels. Usually insurers demand a certain level of quality and market position to be successful. The benefits of negotiation can be fairly dramatic. In one upstate New York community, a range of specialists who formed a large, health system–aligned IPA are able to receive reimbursement from managed care companies at approximately 140 percent of the Medicare fee schedule, compared to other private practice physicians who receive 110 to 115 percent.

INCENTIVES FOR THE ACADEMIC MEDICAL CENTER

Academic medical centers have created their own unique incentives to motivate participation in medical staff organizations. The medical staff of academic medical centers is usually employed through a wholly integrated faculty practice plan, which hires faculty, establishes compensation, and oversees the pursuit of tenure (or other) employment status (e.g., contractual relationships with physicians, clinical/nontenure tracks, etc.).

Incentives for participation in the academic medical center medical staff organization are unique and rarely applicable to most community hospitals systems. In academic medical centers, physician alignment is already significant and accomplished, unlike in the community hospital setting. Some of the powerful incentives that academic medical centers provide include market leverage; prestige; ability to pursue academic (particularly research and teaching) endeavors within the wide latitude of freedom allowed through the general academic environment, and specifically the tenure structure; and the halo effect of affiliation with high-quality institutions.

DETERMINING WHAT INCENTIVES TO OFFER

How should a hospital determine the highest priorities to offer as incentives? A good practice outreach program (described in Chapter 6) is a start. Also, a periodic medical staff survey can help organizations gather market intelligence and determine physician perspectives on what is expected from medical staff membership.

In particular, hospitals and systems must give thoughtful consideration and seek legal counsel to determine how incentives for active participation on the medical staff can be accomplished within the confines of regulatory constraints and precedent-setting legal cases.

By participating in hospital or system initiatives, the physician should achieve the same or similar economic benefits as would occur if the physician, in partnership with an independent developer, pulled ancillaries out of the hospital setting. Economic incentives do not imply payments or subsidies to physicians. The lessons of the late 1980s and early 1990s pointed out the fallacies of practice acquisition and employment of primary care physicians. The benefit to physicians should be the ability to be a viable independent, affiliated physician practice, and participation in a medical staff organization should offer demonstrable benefits—whether they be economic or otherwise.

REFERENCES

Afable, R. 2003. Personal interview, July 28.

Benko, L. 2003. "Get Doctors Opinion." *Modern Healthcare* 33 (24): 18.

Brogadir, S. 2003. Personal interview, July 16.

Brideau, L. 2003. Personal interview, July 16.

Coile, R. C., Jr. 2003. *Futurescan 2003: A Forecast of Healthcare Trends 2003–2007.* Chicago: Health Administration Press.

Demby, E. H. 1991. "Advertising Is Not a Panacea for Physicians." *Marketing News*, November 25, 4.

Fong, T. 2003. "Not Making the Grade." *Modern Healthcare* 33 (22): 12.

Glaser, L. 2003. Personal interview, July 28.

Health Care Advisory Board. 1999. *The Physician Perspective—Understanding the Basis of Physician Facility Selection (and Defection).* Washington, DC: Health Care Advisory Board.

Health Management Technology. 2003. "Easy Access." *Health Management Technology* 24 (4): 45.

Health News Digest. 2003. "Hospitalists Taking Care of Patients." [Online article; retrieved 11/19/03.] http://www.healthnewsdigest.com/news/hlth_hospitalists-2 .html.

Holder, L., and A. Cochran. 2003. "Recovering Physician Loyalty." *Healthcare Executive* 18 (2): 65.

Jackson, C. 2001. "Doctors Find Hospitalists Save Time and Money." *American Medical News* 44 (7): 1.

Kinyon, C. C. 2003. "One CFO's Success with Transitioning to an Automated Patient Record." *Healthcare Financial Management* 57 (2): 52–56.

Kuperman, G., and R. Gibson. 2003. "Computer Physician Order Entry: Benefits, Costs, and Issues." *Annals of Internal Medicine* 139 (1): 31–39.

Maguire, P. 2001. "Despite Their Booming Numbers, Hospitalists Face Growing Pain." *ACP-ASIM Observer* [Online article; retrieved 11/20/03.] http://www.acponline.org/journals/news/May01/hospitalists.htm.

McGinley, L. 2003. "Merit Pay for Top Hospitals—Medicare Plan Would Give Bonuses for Superior Care; Tracking Hip Surgery Results." *Wall Street Journal*, May 27, D1.

Messinger, S., and T. Welter. 2003. "Today's Key Drivers of Physician Loyalty." *Healthcare Financial Management* 57 (5): 78–82.

Rovinsky, M. 2002. "Physician Input: A Critical Strategic-Planning Tool." *Healthcare Financial Management* 56 (1): 36–38.

Smith, D. 2003. Personal interview, December 7.

Solovy, A. 2002. "Most Wired 2002: Health Care's Technology Leaders." *Trustee* 55 (9): 30–32.

Wachter, R., and L. Goldman. 2002. "The Hospitalist Movement 5 Years Later." *Journal of the American Medical Association* 287 (4): 487.

Wright, R. 2003. Personal interview, July 28.

CHAPTER 5

Competitive Strategies
for a Hostile Market

WHEN PHYSICIAN RELATIONSHIPS deteriorate or become acrimonious, how can medical staff organizations implement strategies to compete effectively against nonaligned physicians, independent developers, and niche specialty providers from outside the community who are not committed to the medical staff organization's viability? When incentives, such as those discussed in Chapter 4, fail to motivate physicians to be on the active staff of a hospital, and other attempts to work with physicians and address their concerns have failed, unfortunately (from the standpoint of use of community resources) competitive strategies are often employed.

OPTIONS FOR PHYSICIANS

When the relationship is one of separatism and competition, physicians who were formerly aligned with a hospital can become capable and formidable competitors. The manifestations of a competitive relationship may include the following:

- Development of a freestanding, service line–specific hospital, such as a heart hospital or orthopedic hospital
- Development of an independent ambulatory surgery center with or without hospital ownership participation
- Development of independent imaging or other ambulatory diagnostic or treatment services (e.g., cardiac diagnostics, dermatology, or plastic surgery procedures)

Physicians may also just withdraw from the hospital environment and formal structures. Ophthalmologists, gastroenterologists, and those specialists who work entirely or almost entirely in the ambulatory setting commonly practice in an environment far removed from the hospital setting. These practitioners may work exclusively in their office, an ambulatory surgery center, or a diagnostic and treatment center.

If the market situation becomes contentious and no options for repairing hospital-physician relationships are apparent, physicians may choose to pursue one of the courses of action discussed in the following paragraphs:

1. Align with another compatible hospital and shift cases and referrals elsewhere. Aligning with another hospital may be successful in some markets, and it may help physicians work through feelings of vengeance, but this strategy can also backfire. In the case of a 10-physician independent orthopedic practice in upstate New York that was historically aligned with a healthcare system, the physicians were perturbed when a 140-physician multispecialty group that was closely aligned with the healthcare system began to recruit additional orthopedic surgeons. In response, the independent orthopedic practice shifted surgical procedures and inpatient admissions to the other hospital in the market. In this situation, each party is likely to be a loser.

The recruitment efforts of the large, multispecialty group will eventually create an excess number of orthopedic surgeons for the declining population, which is not likely to increase to accommodate the excess existing orthopedic surgery supply. Exacerbating the situation is the possibility that the competitor hospital may build additional surgery capacity, perhaps even a joint venture ambulatory surgery center with the private practice orthopedic group, in a market that is already well served.

2. Strip high-margin services out of the hospital. In a competitive situation involving a hospital and physicians, one of the likely courses of action is for a physician practice to provide diagnostic and treatment services in the group practice setting, instead of relying on the provision of services at the hospital.

According to Lou Glaser, Esq. (2003), the regulatory environment in many respects encourages this outmigration into a group practice by allowing flexibility under physician anti-self-referral laws that generally permit the provision of in-office ancillary services. However, approximately 50 percent of states rely on certificate-of-need regulations, which may be an impediment to providing diagnostic and treatment services in a physician practice.

Prevalent examples of stripping diagnostic and treatment services are imaging by radiologists, primary care physicians, and orthopedic surgeons; outpatient surgery by ophthalmologists, otorhinolaryngologists, orthopedic surgeons, general surgeons, plastic surgeons, and others performing primarily ambulatory procedures; cardiac diagnostics by cardiologists; and endoscopy by gastroenterologists. Physicians who provide in-office ancillary services are motivated to do so by lucrative financial opportunities. Data from the Medical Group Management Association demonstrate that physicians who have ancillaries in their practice make on average 20 to 30 percent more than physicians who do not (MGMA 2003).

3. Compete with the hospital by providing incentives to office staff. Because physicians are generally classified as for-profit professional corporations, they have more flexibility to provide creative employee reward systems because they are unencumbered by the regulatory environment constraining not-for-profit hospitals and the potential loss of not-for-profit status. Staff incentive programs include offering bonus payments to employees for achieving bottom-line targets or sharing a percentage of cost savings.

Hospitals are catching up and becoming very creative in the area of nonphysician staff retention incentives.

4. Build and cultivate referral relationships. If a cardiac surgeon would like to maintain strong clinical referral relationships with cardiologists, the surgeon cultivates those relationships. A hospital need not enter into this dynamic. Examples of techniques physicians use range from grand rounds case presentations to the demonstration of clinical skills and expertise to building strong personal relationships. These strong physician-to-physician links can preclude a hospital from pursuing other choices for surgical services. Specialists can also cultivate clinical and personal relationships with primary care physicians in an effort to solidify referral relationships.

HOSPITAL AND SYSTEM OPTIONS

When relationships with physicians are severed, a hospital may choose to pursue competitive strategies. In these cases, a hospital carefully considers a long list of options and tailors their strategy to accommodate unique situations and particular practice characteristics. These strategies may permanently sever or seriously damage any future relationship with the physicians involved, so they should be employed with caution.

1. Make credentialing decisions based on conflicts of interest. This credentialing strategy has received quite a bit of attention recently with the proliferation of competitive initiatives by physicians. One understandable potential course of action by hospitals is to sever all relationships with physician practices that launch initiatives that place them in direct competition with the hospital. A hospital may terminate or curtail hospital credentials and privileges, which allow access to hospital facilities and services. Some physicians would ask, "So what?" Many physicians perceive that the only reward for being on a medical staff is being required to attend many, many meetings; however, exclusion from a medical staff can have implications for referral relationships and access to managed care contracts.

Maine is a battleground for these types of initiatives. The 560-bed Maine Medical Center developed a heart hospital in Portland, which competes with Central Maine Medical Center's heart center. Central Maine mandated that cardiologists would have to sign a contract stating they would not work anywhere else, and it cut ties to any cardiologist affiliated with the Maine Medical Center's competing heart hospital nearby (Duff 2002). Central Maine followed a path chosen by an increasing number of hospitals: signing exclusive contracts with certain specialists and limiting or denying privileges to physicians on the staffs of competing institutions (Terry 2002).

According to Lou Glaser, Esq., "Obviously, these types of actions raise legal issues, particularly antitrust concerns. To date, most courts have sided with hospitals that have restricted privileges or medical staff membership of physicians who own competing facilities. Nonetheless, hospitals that pursue these hardball tactics should do so carefully. A hospital's motivation should not be based on a desire to harm competition, because the law views competition as beneficial" (Glaser 2003).

Some hospitals consider establishing minimum encounter levels to attain active medical staff membership eligibility. According to Linda Haddad (2003) of Horty Springer, & Mattern,

> We do not recommend a number of minimum contacts because we fear the anti-kickback enforcers. Rather, we recommend that in certain specialties, a physician be required to use our facility as his/her primary facility. It is nearly impossible to measure, but it emphasizes that the hospital is not a way station and it is not to be used solely to accommodate nonpaying or expensive patients. Plus it requires adequate activity to evaluate competence and to learn one's way around the hospital and personnel to be able to serve patients more effectively.

2. Grant active staff credentials for good citizenship. This strategy of rewarding good citizenship is related to the concept of credentialing based on conflicts of interest, but it focuses on establishing policies and procedures for granting or denying active medical staff privileges when physicians pursue initiatives not in the best interest of the hospital. One hospital chief executive officer located in the Mid-Atlantic states struggles with pressure to adopt a policy of granting medical staff credentials to physicians with potentially competitive behavior:

> We are faced with our cardiology specialists making moves to compete with the hospital on all of our outpatient cardiology services. They are the only cardiologists in town and are good clinicians and have been loyal to the hospital for years. One of the physicians is on the board. Our legal counsel (a very highly regarded national firm) has urged us to take two steps: remove the physician from the board due to his conflict of interest and have the board adopt a very strong policy defining one critical element of "good citizenship" for remaining on the medical staff as supporting the economic health of the hospital, meaning that you don't compete directly with the hospital on these sort of important services.

Legally, these types of actions can be perceived as potentially anticompetitive, according to Lou Glaser, Esq. (2003): "It is important to be aware that the OIG [Office of Inspector General] is examining the issue of whether the granting of privileges constitutes remuneration for purposes of the anti-kickback statute. In other words, if only physicians who are good and admit patients are granted privileges, are they really being given a kickback? The timing issue is really related to whether a hospital can articulate a good reason for taking the action short of trying to hurt a competitor."

3. Disenfranchise competing practices by excluding them from payer contracts. Physicians who are employed or formally aligned with hospitals and systems typically benefit from favorable third-party payer payments that are not available to their independent private practice physician colleagues. A hospital or system usually has the clout and market presence to negotiate more firmly with payers. In the example cited earlier, in one upstate New York community, private practice physicians have negotiated payments from commercial payers representing 110 to 115 percent of the Medicare fee schedule. A large, hospital-aligned, multispecialty group practice in the same community benefits from more favorable reimbursement of more than 140 percent of the Medicare fee schedule from the same commercial payers.

According to Rick Afable, M.D. (2003), "Hospitals are often the biggest employers and wield significant leverage in determining which employees can receive care." An example of this strategy occurred in suburban Phoenix. A two-hospital healthcare system, faced with a potential competitive threat from an independent specialty niche hospital, informed physician participants in the competitive venture that the niche hospital would not necessarily be eligible for participation as a service provider on the health system's managed care plan. A total of 30,000 members of the managed care plan would be affected by this new rule. The physicians aligning themselves with the specialty niche hospital could potentially be precluded from accessing a large portion of business because those patients who were covered with the health system's managed care product could not be covered by their insurance plan for services provided at the independent specialty hospital. In addition to potential exclusion from payer contracts, the physicians were threatened with potential loss of medical staff privileges. Each of these threats contributed to a decline in physician interest, and the independent surgical hospital developer abandoned the market.

4. Restrict the network. For those hospitals that still own some or all of a managed care plan, the hospital can require the use of hospital-owned or affiliated sites and services, particularly for hospital and health system employees. A competitive entity, such as a physician-owned ambulatory surgery center, would not qualify. This strategy can be particularly effective if payers and employers agree to restrict the provision of services to certain providers.

5. Foster competitive recruitment. Physician practices on a medical staff are often competitive with one another. A hospital can foster further competition by helping more closely aligned practices with physician recruitment. In the case of a suburban Philadelphia hospital, two cardiology practices have become both competitive and complacent with the hospital. Competition manifests itself by the existing groups adding a comprehensive array of cardiac services in their offices, including EKGs, echocardiography, stress testing, Holter monitoring, and nuclear imaging studies. Service levels provided by these physicians (e.g., service to unassigned emergency department [ED] cases and response time for subspecialty consults to other services) are viewed to be inadequate by other physicians on the medical staff. The hospital's strategy is to pursue the recruitment of a competitive cardiology practice and grant this competitive practice access to reading cardiac diagnostic services in the hospital, participation in ED call coverage (to build practice volume through unassigned call patients), and the opportunity to compete with the existing groups for clinical referrals.

6. *Refuse to provide a transfer agreement.* In many states, to gain state licensure, niche specialty hospitals and ambulatory care centers must execute formal transfer agreements to acute healthcare facilities should cases require more acute intervention. A good example is a formal transfer agreement between a freestanding, physician-owned, ambulatory surgery center and a hospital's emergency department, back-up intensive care unit, and inpatient beds, should an untoward clinical event or episode occur. A hospital could refuse to execute a formal transfer agreement between a freestanding, physician-owned, ambulatory surgery center and the hospital's emergency department, intensive care unit, and inpatient beds.

7. *Promote price competition.* A hospital or system may discount prices to insurers for services provided by a competitor, such as a specialty niche hospital or ambulatory surgery center. In this situation, a hospital or system will decide to provide more favorable rates to payers to earn their business.

8. *Offer retention bonuses to nurses and other valuable technical staff.* Retention programs may be sufficient incentive to prevent the loss of staff to a competitor, such as a for-profit specialty hospital.

In some cases, retention bonuses are structured with higher payments in later years to ensure a more significant, long-term commitment. For example, payments can be made over a five-year period, with $1,000 in year one, followed by annual payments of $3,000, $5,000, $7,000, and $9,000.

9. Strengthen strategic alignments with loyal, noncompetitive practices. In some cases, physicians who are closely aligned with, rather than competitive with, a healthcare organization are made eligible for joint ventures, management contracts, and other formal business relationships with the hospital or system. In other instances, hospitals foster strong referral relationships among loyal physician practices.

10. Facilitate practice promotion and marketing. As discussed in Chapter 4, hospitals may have a unique opportunity to help aligned physicians promote and market their practices. Examples might include participation in a hospital telephone and web site direct linkage referral program, involvement in other promotional initiatives (e.g., brochures, yellow pages, etc.), and access to ED call coverage, which may be an important vehicle for accessing unassigned patients.

11. Rouse community pressure. In one rural Northeast community, hospital-aligned physicians planned to open an independent ambulatory surgery center. Through a letter-writing campaign to the local newspaper, hospital management was able to exert sufficient community pressure, which one physician said manifested itself as "shame and guilt," resulting in the physicians abandoning their plans.

12. Create doubt. By casting the regulatory or reimbursement environment as uncertain, or discrediting another potential partner, especially one that does not have a good track record of working in a collaborative manner in a community, hospital leaders can engage in a "doubt raising" campaign. Components may include a letter-writing campaign and discrediting financials. One four-hospital system in the metropolitan Boston market found this to be an effective strategy. Managers of the Boston-area system pointed out that taxes were not factored into a developer's financial pro formas, nor were start-up costs, realistic market-based utilization forecasts, or reasonable expense assumptions.

13. Consider advocacy efforts. In some cases, not-for-profit community hospitals expend a fair amount of energy working with state and national legislative bodies to change the laws that allow physician investment in specialty hospitals and surgery centers. Many credit the American Hospital Association's lobbying efforts with the recent 18-month federal moratorium on specialty hospital development.

CONCLUSION

Exploring all opportunities to work amiably with physicians, gain their trust, and promote active involvement on a medical staff organization should be explored before hospitals and systems employ strategies to thwart competitive physician initiatives. The community benefit of collaboration can be tremendous. But hospitals and systems cannot sit idly by as physicians strip away valuable services that enable hospitals to remain full-service healthcare providers for a defined community. Competitive strategies, therefore, must be considered as possible approaches for ensuring the future viability of hospitals and systems. More detailed information on competitive strategy is presented in Zuckerman's (2003) *Improve Your Competitive Strategy.*

REFERENCES

Afable, R. 2003. Personal interview, July 28.

Duff, S. 2002. "Change of Heart." *Modern Healthcare* 32 (14): 18.

Glaser, L. 2003. Personal interview, August 13.

Haddad, L. 2003. Personal interview, July 30.

Medical Group Management Association. 2003. *Physician Compensation and Production Survey: 2003 Report Based on 2002 Data.* Englewood, CO: MGMA.

Terry, K. 2002. "Hospital Hardball." *Medical Economics* 79 (15): 72–81.

Zuckerman, A. 2003. *Improve Your Competitive Strategy: A Guide for the Healthcare Executive.* Chicago: Health Administration Press

CHAPTER 6

Techniques to Foster Effective Working Relationships

NUMEROUS TECHNIQUES CAN foster productive and positive working relationships between hospital management and physicians on the medical staff. Using these techniques as a guide for everyday dealings with the medical staff, hospitals and systems can begin to forge a foundation of mutual trust with physicians and earn their loyalty. Such loyalty may create opportunities to transition physician relationships from independence and competition to more collaborative dealings and more active participation on medical staff organizations.

Not all of the techniques discussed in this chapter will apply to all situations, and most will need to be tailored to account for unique circumstances. According to Leo Brideau, FACHE, president and chief executive officer of the Columbia St. Mary's Health System in Milwaukee, Wisconsin, an important prerequisite to the consideration of any of these techniques is to recognize that the hospital environment and the physician practice environment are different (Brideau 2003). Applying this mindset will help hospital management and physicians appreciate and respect that each is working with different cultural and educational backgrounds and viewing healthcare delivery and its environmental influences from very divergent perspectives.

Differences in Decision Making

Physicians work in predominantly entrepreneurial environments; hospital leaders usually work in environments that tend to be bureaucratic, garnering input from many constituents potentially affected by a decision. The bureaucratic hospital management setting often demands exhaustive analysis to reach consensus on issues, compared to the rapid, independent decision making in physician practices. The bureaucratic hospital environment is also viewed as more conservative and thorough in decision making. Boards of trustees today typically establish an environment for prudent and methodical decision making, a culture and attitude that can be viewed as onerous by the physician operating in an entrepreneurial environment.

According to Robert Pickoff, M.D., "to be fair, it is more than bureaucracy that leads to exhaustive analysis on the hospital side …there are allocation of cost issues that aren't considered in a physician's office mostly because physicians are ignorant of many of these issues. Educating physicians about the issues a hospital or system considers important is another good technique" (Pickoff 2003).

Personal Investment

Often overlooked in physician-hospital dynamics is the issue of physicians' personal stake in business dealings. When economic relationships are on the table, healthcare executives have inherently lower stakes because they are negotiating the investment of organizational funds. Physicians on a medical staff who choose to participate in an economic relationship with a hospital or system are contemplating the use of personal funds. For a physician, such initiatives may require them to draw down a personal bank account, take out a second mortgage, or borrow from a bank or venture capitalist. The capitalization of a joint venture may compete with the need for college funds for children or house-renovation money; hospital managers do not have to personally invest in these initiatives.

These differences in personal investment and decision making add up to enormous potential for misunderstanding on both sides. Clearly, the environments in which hospital leaders and physicians operate are quite different, and as a result, each party's perspective can be shaped differently. Nevertheless, the techniques in this chapter present some common ground for forging effective and mutually beneficial ties between physicians and the hospital that will strengthen medical staff organizations.

TECHNIQUE 1: DON'T FIGHT THE INEVITABLE OUTMIGRATION OF ANCILLARY SERVICES AND TECHNICAL FEES

Hospital and system leaders can be short sighted when considering how to respond to the increasingly prevalent provision of ambulatory services out of the hospital environment. Some leaders battle ferociously to retain all outpatient services in the hospital setting. But this movement of services out of the hospital setting is neither new nor unexpected and is becoming more common (see Figure 6.1 for more detail on this trend).

Several issues drive this trend, including the following:

- Physicians are motivated by stagnation, or in some cases reduction, in their professional fee schedules. Essentially, physicians are working harder for the same or less money, as shown in Figure 6.2.

Figure 6.1. Outmigration of Ancillary Services

Outpatient Service Line	Site of Care	1994	2001
Gastroenterology	Freestanding	19	36
	Hospital based	81	64
Urology	Freestanding	16	30
	Hospital based	84	70
Neurology	Freestanding	11	24
	Hospital based	89	76
Ear, Nose, and Throat	Freestanding	17	27
	Hospital based	83	73
Dermatology	Freestanding	27	35
	Hospital based	73	65
Orthopedics	Freestanding	26	36
	Hospital based	74	64
Ophthalmology	Freestanding	56	68
	Hospital based	44	32

Source: Excerpted from Coile (2003).

- Physicians are also motivated by escalating practice costs. The combination of stagnant reimbursement and escalating expenses has a double effect, causing a deterioration of take-home compensation by physicians, as detailed in Figure 6.3.
- Technological advancements will continue to drive care into the outpatient setting. Technologies used for diagnosis and treatment will continue to evolve and become less invasive, smaller, more cost-effective, and generally more suitable for physician offices. Examples abound in surgery, chemotherapy, endoscopy, erdoscopy, and other routine outpatient diagnostic and treatment services.
- The elimination of state certificate-of-need regulations as a barrier to market entry is making it easier for physicians to provide services that were traditionally provided exclusively in hospitals. Approximately one-half of all states still maintain certificate-of-need regulations, which restrict open-market

Figure 6.2. Percent Change in Compensation Adjusted for Inflation Compared to Change in Utilization, 1996–2002

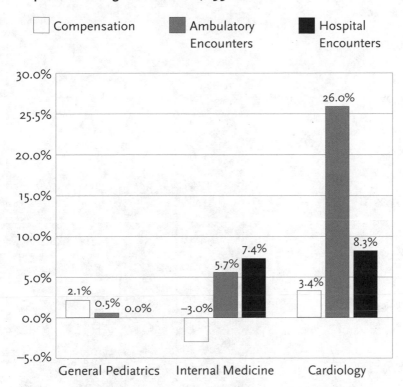

☐ Compensation   ▓ Ambulatory Encounters   ■ Hospital Encounters

Note: Comparison year is 2002.

Sources: MGMA (1997, 2003). Used with permission from the Medical Group Management Association, 104 Inverness Terrace East, Englewood, CO, 80112-5306; 303/799-1111. www.mgma.com.

program and service development by establishing a process that attempts to rationalize community resources.

- For-profit partners are facilitating the outmigration of ancillary services. In ambulatory surgery, no less than 50 for-profit, publicly traded companies are interested in partnering with physicians to develop ambulatory surgery centers (Health Strategies & Solutions, Inc. 2003). Many companies cite operational efficiency, management expertise, contracting

Figure 6.3. Percent Change in Physician Compensation Compared to Percent Changes in Typical Practice Costs Adjusted for Inflation, 1996–2002

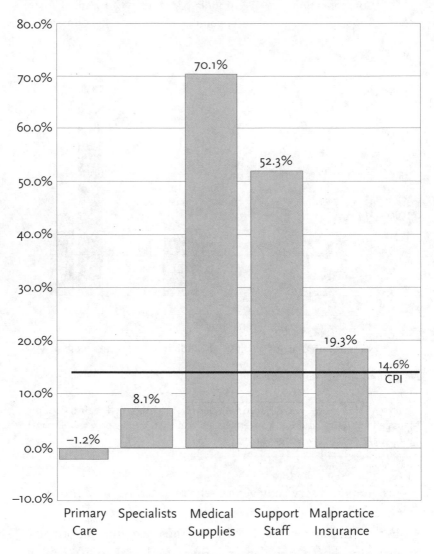

Note: Comparison year is 2002.

Sources: MGMA (1997, 2003); InflationData.com (2004). MGMA data are used with permission from the Medical Group Management Association, 104 Inverness Terrace East, Englewood, CO, 80112-5306; 303/799-1111. www. mgma.com.

capabilities, and most importantly, access to capital as reasons for a partnership with a for-profit company.

According to Robert Pickoff, M.D., "Rather than fighting this inevitable outmigration of services, one obvious alternative for hospitals to pursue is to partner with physicians to salvage a portion of ambulatory services. Physicians may welcome the deep investor pockets of the hospital in return for a piece of the action, even a 51 percent share" (Pickoff 2003).

The lesson of this issue is that in some cases, hospital management should focus energies on those healthcare services not likely to be moved out of the traditional hospital environment. In other cases, management will need to focus on services to backfill or replace those services that outmigrate. In yet other cases, hospitals will find it appropriate to partner or compete with physicians in the provision of redundant healthcare services. The course of action will depend on the specifics of the situation, including the healthcare service, the physician practice, and hospital capabilities. Getting started on this topic is reviewed in Chapter 7.

TECHNIQUE 2: DON'T UNDERESTIMATE PROCESS REQUIREMENTS

Creating a viable, strong, and effective medical staff organization requires a substantial expenditure of time, money, and effort. Hospitals have a long track record of failed collaboration efforts, which has generated animosity and even outright hostility among physicians. According to a vice president of a Mid-Atlantic health system, new and more effective dealings with physicians will take "ten times the effort you plan in your day planner." Physician practices are still typically small groups, and each will require interaction and explanation of initiatives underway or contemplated.

Delegating the day-to-day responsibility for negotiating arrangements with physicians entirely to middle managers is short sighted and inappropriate; not only does this approach tend to delay the process because of the "I will get back to you with approval" mentality, but it demonstrates insufficient and insincere commitment to the importance of these relationships.

TECHNIQUE 3: IMPROVE HOSPITAL OPERATIONS EFFICIENCY

Improving hospital efficiency is an important technique for building effective relationships with physicians. High-priority operations and systems improvements and the demonstration of efficiency should address, at a minimum, the following:

- Ancillary procedure and test scheduling: access and convenience
- Patient information; results reporting: turnaround time, electronic 24/7 access, and accuracy
- Operating room performance: utilization, hours of operation, room turnaround time, and staffing
- Wait times for different patient cohorts (e.g., urgent, emergent, and nonurgent) and specialist coverage in the emergency department
- Provision of hospitalists for inpatient coverage
- Average length of stay
- Cost per case data
- Clinical outcomes measures and results

TECHNIQUE 4: DEVELOP A FORMAL PHYSICIAN RELATIONSHIP OR "OUTREACH" PROGRAM

Physician outreach programs were commonplace 25 years ago. However, with the Balanced Budget Act financial pressures and increased efforts by pharmaceutical sales representatives to maximize personal visits to practices most of these programs have been severely curtailed or discontinued or are difficult to differentiate from the efforts of pharmaceutical representatives.

Seasoned managers, executives, and board members may question the value of physician relationship programs, especially at a time when budget items such as strategic planning and marketing are being scrutinized to demonstrate their worth as measured by a very short time frame. However, many hospitals and systems are realizing that they can substantially increase market share in target service lines and geographic areas as a direct result of activating an organized process for seeking physician input and then aggressively addressing physician concerns. For most hospitals and systems, the cost of operating a comprehensive physician outreach program may be far less than the expense of major defections from the medical staff. Further, the outreach efforts of competitive hospitals to physicians historically loyal to your medical staff can be easily but disastrously overlooked.

Successful outreach programs should do the following:

- Monitor physician activity levels at the hospital and its affiliated sites, using monthly (at a minimum) encounter data for admissions, procedures, and other encounters and referrals
- Target top-tier (e.g., the top five to ten percent of active or potentially active) physicians to be included in an outreach program
- Track substantial changes in activity levels (e.g., an increase or decrease of 20 percent) every month; reasons for changes in activity may be as simple as vacation time, but may also be a result of substantial dissatisfaction with emergency department coverage, staff coverage on inpatient units, or operating room procedures
- Establish a formal system for practice visits to ascertain impediments to high satisfaction levels with hospital services
- Address and monitor issues that are raised by physicians and report back to physicians promptly on actions to be undertaken

- Devote senior management time and energy to outreach rather than delegate the responsibility to sales representatives

One healthcare system in the Midwest devotes two to three full-time staff members to this effort: 2.5 FTEs. Three of five workdays are spent on the road meeting with physicians, averaging five appointments per day. This effort adds up to 40 physician visits per week or approximately 2,000 individual physician visits per year—visits that take place in the physician office, on their turf, listening to their issues. The remainder of dedicated staff time is spent addressing and remedying any unresolved physician issues. Three potential responses to physicians' concerns are communicated: "The issue is fixed, and this is how"; "The issue will be fixed by the following date, and in this manner"; or "Here is why we cannot fix the issue, but we will reexamine the issue by the following date."

TECHNIQUE 5: BALANCE CONSISTENCY WITH FLEXIBILITY

Overall guidelines and principles for collaboration are useful as are clear evaluation criteria to determine whether partnership or competitive relationships with members of a hospital's medical staff are more advantagous. Developing guidelines provides a context for each potential arrangement and helps hospital administrators avoid the perception that they make special and unique sweetheart deals with individual practices. Example guidelines and evaluation criteria are described in Chapter 7. Such guidelines help hospitals maintain a consistent, objective, and fair approach to collaborative relationships with physicians. However, hospitals and systems must avoid coming to the negotiating table with rigid expectations for physician relationships or "all or nothing" demands. The failed physician-hospital relationships of the 1990s are evidence that this "my way or the highway" or "one size fits all" mentality is not acceptable to physicians and fails to enable physicians to have meaningful and valued input into key decisions about healthcare delivery.

TECHNIQUE 6: REPRESENT COLLABORATION BETWEEN HOSPITAL AND MEDICAL STAFF AS A BINDING AND LONG-TERM COMMITMENT

The early models of physician-hospital partnerships suffered from the mere fact that they were highly experimental. The partnerships also fell victim to unrealistic expectations about joining together such diverse groups and motivating physicians to buy into the value of and need for partnerships. Many physician-hospital relationships were initiated during the flurry of activity associated with the perceived need to develop tightly bound integrated delivery networks in the late 1980s and throughout the 1990s to assume full-risk capitation contracts. One physician leader in a New England hospital system accused hospitals of a "bullying, thug mentality" when observing regional hospitals' efforts to impose organization to hospital-physician partnerships.

To avoid committing similar mistakes in the future, physicians, hospitals, and systems need to adopt the perspective that "We're in this together, for the long haul." Storms will be weathered, and together we will find meaningful ways to collaborate that will be beneficial to ourselves and the community we serve.

Successful (and long-lasting) business relationships formally develop a business plan. Previously, in the absence of formal business plans, faulty assumptions characterized business relationships between hospitals and physicians, including misconceptions that:

- Physicians and hospitals could rationally divide up a shrinking reimbursement pool from physician-hospital organizations in the form of capitated or global fee payments.

- Physicians and hospitals could measure and monitor utilization of healthcare services to work successfully under capitation or other risk arrangements.
- Hospitals could employ physicians and instill the same entrepreneurial spirit and accountability as demonstrated by physicians who are in private practice.

TECHNIQUE 7: INVOLVE PHYSICIANS IN HOSPITAL LEADERSHIP

According to Michael Rovinsky (2002),

> The inability of IDSs to align physicians' interests with those of the organization has been due in large part to a failure to develop governance and strategic-planning structures that adequately incorporate physicians' perspectives. Physician input into the strategic development of these organizations often was limited to formal or informal "confidential stakeholder" interviews with key physician leaders identified by the hospital or health system administration. Occasionally, select physicians would be invited to participate in a strategic planning retreat, or results and recommendations from the strategic planning process would be presented to a "physician advisory group" that was formed to serve as a vehicle for physician input. But these tactics were insufficient to foster physician support of the organization's business strategy and goals.

Except in unusual circumstances, physician input into hospital and system management issues has been restricted to clinical care. As hospitals and physicians become more equal partners in the healthcare delivery system, physicians must participate more fully in crucial strategic and financial decision making so that all parties understand the potential risks and rewards of future actions. When physician-hospital relationships demonstrate a spirit of partnership, cooperation, and collaboration and a willingness to share control and work together to face strategic issues, more successful outcomes are ensured for both physicians and hospitals.

Hospitals should strive to include physician leaders in both formal and informal capacities. Formal leadership positions, not figurehead slots, must be formed. Formal and informal forums for candid discussion and truth telling must be created.

For the Columbia St. Mary's Health System, Leo Brideau includes physicians in leadership, but also actively solicits physician input on major decisions made by the system. For example, more than 70 physicians provided input into a recent strategic planning initiative. Columbia St. Mary's also formed a physician advisory group to provide input into critical program and service developments, such as program planning for a new replacement hospital in downtown Milwaukee. In addition, in the Columbia St. Mary's cancer program planning initiative, every physician related in some fashion to oncology services was invited to participate in the process of determining the future direction of oncology services. Brideau's general philosophy is that physicians can opt out of program and service line planning (and other planning initiatives), but his goal is to not allow the physicians aligned with Columbia St. Mary's to feel left out of these important planning processes (Brideau 2003).

Including young physicians in leadership initiatives is critical. Competing responsibilities and priorities might get in the way, but solidify the involvement of physicians as early as possible. Compensate physicians for time spent in these planning and leadership roles if necessary; compensation may be a better option than leaving out this important constituency.

Particularly critical to gaining the trust and commitment of younger physicians is the understanding that most business dealings with physicians and hospital management should be conducted and resolved outside of the medical executive committee. Business is better conducted in settings that are comfortable for physicians, such as in the medical staff lounge or at the country club on weekends.

Some hospitals and systems elevate the lead administrative physician role on the management team by appointing a chief medical officer. This role often includes managing information systems and quality and outcomes initiatives (in addition to fostering productive relationships with the medical staff), in contrast to the perceived less influential role of vice president of medical affairs. Many physician executives plan to pursue hospital chief medical officer roles in the future.

One way to maximize participation in leadership is to establish term limits for physician leaders. For example, allow a physician leader to serve an elected term for two or three years, after which the physician is ineligible to serve for a certain period of time.

The Bristol Group has established recommended targets for physician participation in hospital leadership: 30 percent of the hospital board of trustees and 50 percent of strategic planning committees are expected to be physicians. Whether or not these proportions are appropriate for a hospital or system depends on the particular situation; the goal is more physician involvement in hospital management (Sherer 1999).

TECHNIQUE 8: DEMONSTRATE THE VALUE OF ANY FORMAL COLLABORATION

The value of a physician-hospital relationship can be expressed as direct financial contribution or return on investment to each of the parties in the partnership, or as indirect value, measured, for example, by elimination of the "hassle factor" or by strategic importance. Other successful collaborative initiatives have demonstrated the value in seeking early gains in the pursuit of formal business relationships with physicians to gain momentum for other potential arrangements with physicians.

Past collaborations between physicians and hospitals failed to provide accurate and timely financial and utilization performance monitoring. Instead, financial forecasts and utilization projections were made, but ongoing monitoring was usually nonexistent. Today, financial benefits to each party, including hospitals, physicians, and third party developers or investors, must be monitored and demonstrated. Examples of performance indicators that can be used to demonstrate financial performance are outcomes and other quality-of-care measures, patient satisfaction, return on investment, net income, profit, volume indicators, and market share.

Generally, efforts to collaborate with physicians focus on financial benefit, but hospitals can offer other meaningful benefits, such as operating room block scheduling and facilities located near physician offices.

TECHNIQUE 9: AVOID MEETING WITH PHYSICIANS IN THE EXECUTIVE SUITE

New management teams should make every effort to meet physicians on their own turf. The new chief executive officer of a Philadelphia health system put many miles on his car recently while employing this strategy, but, as one private practice physician put it, "at least he [was] out of the corporate palace." By visiting physicians in their offices, hospital managers and executives demonstrate their understanding of the value of a physician's time and show a willingness to become acquainted with physicians on a more personal level. This situation also applies to senior management assuming a greater role in practice outreach on an ongoing basis. In some cases an invitation to the ivory tower demonstrates respect for physician leadership, but more often the executive suite is too formal and intimidating for garnering frank input and fostering healthy dialog.

TECHNIQUE 10: OFFER PHYSICIANS A CHOICE

Many hospital leaders look at physicians as a homogeneous group when in fact physicians are a highly diverse group with wide-ranging perspectives on the type of relationship they want to have with a hospital or system. A one-size-fits-all approach to physician-hospital relationships should be abandoned in favor of more personalized relationships that fit the interests and comfort levels of all categories of physicians: young and old, representatives of solo and group practices, primary care physicians and subspecialists, and community-based and hospital-based physicians.

TECHNIQUE 11: BUILD TRUST AND ENABLE EVOLUTION TO MORE SUBSTANTIAL COLLABORATION

A common theme in past collaboration mistakes was substantial and immediate physician-hospital integration. Many physicians will be more receptive to gradual or phased initiatives that allow trust to be built. If initial success is achieved, a platform of trust will be created, enabling further collaboration.

TECHNIQUE 12: AVOID EXCLUSIVITY AND MEDICAL STAFF SECTION CLOSURE

It is far better to let physicians opt in to potential partnership arrangements than to have the hospital select preferred partners. Hardball strategies may foster an anticompetitive environment and attract the interest of regulators. Fostering competition and choice will hopefully help hospitals avoid a lose-lose outcome—litigation.

TECHNIQUE 13: INVOLVE LEGAL COUNSEL TO AVOID LAND MINES

Systems, hospitals, and physicians must first conceptualize collaboration strategies, business objectives, and services that need to be provided. The possible model or structure can then be constructed to meet the objectives. At this point, legal counsel should scrutinize the feasibility of the plan. By including legal counsel early, the participants can avoid investing significant time and energy in a project or structure that is not legally feasible at the present time or possibly in the future because of likely regulatory changes.

According to Lou Glaser, Esq. (2003), topics that participants should explore in creating arrangements between hospitals and medical staff members include:

- physician anti-self-referral laws (e.g., the "Stark law" and state equivalents)
- state and federal anti-kickback and fraud and abuse laws
- other compliance laws
- federal income tax rules
- tax-exempt bonds
- reasonableness (rather than excessive benefit to physicians)
- certificate-of-need and licensure laws
- corporate practice of medicine laws

TECHNIQUE 14: MONITOR AND COMMUNICATE PERFORMANCE AGAINST EXPECTATIONS

The importance of this technique is best illustrated by observing what happens when performance expectations are not communicated or monitored. Industry performance indicators for employed physicians demonstrate that hospitals and systems typically lose $50,000 to $100,000 per year per physician, yet the oft-stated goal for employed physicians is to operate as close to breakeven as possible.

"Dashboard indicators" of performance are often not developed or not communicated. These dashboard indicators could be developed for many initiatives:

- *Recruitment assistance*: Dashboard indicators include the number of physicians recruited, how many physicians remain in the community after five years, the viability of physician practices, and physician loyalty to a hospital and its specialists.
- *Purchased revenue stream*: Dashboard indicators are collections rate, payer mix, days in accounts receivable, expense levels by major category, and so forth.
- *Competitive situation*: Dashboard indicators include volume of admissions, referrals to specialists, and ancillary services salvaged; competitive recruitment success; financial performance of competitor; and financial performance of medical staff organization.

Performance measures should be developed and measured for both physicians and the hospital.

TECHNIQUE 15: HAVE AN EXIT STRATEGY

Federal and state regulations change almost daily, the reimbursement environment changes frequently, the competitive environment evolves quickly, and individual situations and positions change rapidly. The term or time frame of any major initiatives should allow sufficient time to achieve success, but not be so long as to lock either party into an unwise strategy should the regulatory, reimbursement, or competitive environment change. In addition, the term of any economic partnership should take into account the required capital investment and payback period for the respective venture. Given all the unknowns, agree with physician partners in advance to resyndicate or divest to cut losses if certain key indicators or milestones are not achieved.

CONCLUSION

The success of these techniques will depend heavily on how expertly and creatively they are tailored for the unique situations hospitals and systems face and the level of trust and confidence already present among physician and hospital leaders. Patience, perseverance, and careful planning and monitoring will be key to successfully employing these techniques in building effective working relationships between hospitals and physicians.

REFERENCES

Brideau, L. 2003. Personal interview, July 8.

Coile, R. C., Jr. 2003. *Futurescan 2003: A Forecast of Healthcare Trends: 2003–2007.* Chicago: Health Administration Press.

Glaser, L. 2003. Personal interview, August 13.

Health Strategies & Solutions, Inc. 2003. Company research.

InflationData.com. "Historical CIP." 2004. [Online data; retrieved 1/18/2004.] http://inflationdata.com/Inflation/Consumer_Price_Index/HistoricalCIP.aspx.

Medical Group Management Association. 2003. *Physician Compensation and Production Survey; 2003 Report Based on 2002 Data.* Englewood, CO: MGMA.

————. 2002. *Physician Compensation and Production Survey; 1997 Report Based on 1996 Data.* Englewood, CO: MGMA.

Pickoff, R. 2003. Personal interview, July 8.

Rovinsky, M. 2002. "Physician Input: A Critical Strategic Planning Tool." *Healthcare Financial Management* 56 (1): 36–38.

Sherer, J. L. 1999. "Engaging Physicians in True Strategic Partnership." *Healthcare Executive* 14 (3): 26.

CHAPTER 7

Revitalizing the Medical Staff Organization: How to Get Started

Difficult as it may be to imagine with today's conditions and environment, the medical staff organization of the future will comprise a single hospital or hospital system in more substantial partnership arrangements with loyal, aligned physicians. Evolving to that sort of culture and environment may seem daunting.

After reading the previous six chapters of this book, hospital leaders are likely to ask these questions:

- Where do we start?
- With whom do we partner?
- How do I establish priorities?
- What is the process for categorizing physician practices as potential partners or competitors?

One helpful approach is for hospital management and medical staff leadership to create a continuum to categorize the relationships between the hospital and physicians. On one extreme are "allies," or those with whom to pursue more meaningful relationships, and on the other end are "adversaries" with whom to compete. Physicians may fall somewhere in the middle of the spectrum.

When dealing with the physician adversary/ally continuum, a hospital must determine its ability to sustain both competitive and cooperative physician relationships. According to Richard Afable, M.D. (2003), "Allowing competition and believing in partnerships—both [approaches] cannot coexist in this dysfunctional relationship, in the overall goal of hoping to create a sustained, favorable relationship. One or the other must and will dominate the relationship over time."

As the hospital is sorting out the designations of ally and adversary, physicians will also be increasingly called on to decide the appropriate relationship with hospitals and systems in their community. Their determinations will not be easily made, especially given the numerous misadventures of previous physician-hospital alliances that have damaged hospitals' credibility and trustworthiness.

THE IDEAL ENVIRONMENT FOR CREATING PRINCIPLES OF ALIGNMENT

Many hospitals establish guiding principles for creating and fostering a collaborative environment with physicians. Ideally, these guiding principles should be developed and adopted by the hospital board of trustees, management team, and medical staff during a calm period when the overall environment is collegial. Such an atmosphere engenders clear and objective debate and discussion without focusing on one particular competitive initiative or physician practice. However, if these guiding principles are developed during a time of contentious or even contemptuous relationships, the principles can easily be construed to have anticompetitive, vindictive, or spiteful intent. The likelihood of this situation occurring is particularly strong when the guiding principles lead to more selective and favorable arrangements with some physicians, resulting in preferential treatment and attention or "favored-nation status."

THE CASE FOR GUIDELINES

Guidelines can serve as a starting point for physicians and hospital leaders to establish a context for determining generally whether to pursue collaborative working relationships or whether a competitive posture will be chosen. In most situations, guidelines are endorsed by hospital boards and hospital-affiliated physician organizations (e.g., the medical staff and large affiliated multispecialty groups) and establish parameters for collaborative working relationships.

By failing to develop guidelines such as these, as well as specific partnership evaluation criteria, physicians and hospital leaders are likely react with an "initiative du jour," which is often an initiative that has been applied to a different set of circumstances. Attorneys, accountants, or consultants may also dream up generic initiatives that do not apply to all situations.

Many hospitals establish physician partnership arrangements on the fly. In retrospect, the solutions may prove to be out of context, haphazard, difficult to get out of, and often not objective. Many partnership arrangements are also reactions to unique initiatives, individual personalities and situations, or factors that can be interpreted quite subjectively. Instead, guidelines for collaboration should be created in a proactive manner, not in the heat of the moment, but before the initiative du jour appears on the agenda of the medical executive committee meeting or a senior management strategy session. In each situation, if either body is put into a position of decision making rather than endorsement, the process of collaboration has likely failed.

To suggest that the development of guidelines for collaboration will result in harmony between physicians and the hospital would be naive; typically the strategic objectives of the hospital and its medical staff are clarified in a proactive manner, and the parties are not left in ambiguity about how to respond to a particular situation or initiative. In fact, in many cases the adoption of principles and the evaluation criteria, such as the ones offered in this chapter, lead management and segments of the medical staff to assume a competitive stance.

An example of this development occurred in rural west Texas. A hospital board and its medical staff adopted a set of guiding principles that afforded preferential treatment to orthopedic surgeons. The hospital's major strategic initiative was to build its musculoskeletal service line; the service line lagged other service lines in market share, level of subspecialty depth and breadth, growth, and other factors. In an effort to grow the program, attractive recruitment and retention packages were offered to orthopedic practices that added other physicians. In addition, orthopedic surgeons who contributed their energy to musculoskeletal program development were afforded preferential treatment in advertising and promotional materials (e.g., physician referral lines, hospital brochures, web site linkages, etc.). Eventually, not only general orthopedic surgeons but also orthopedic surgeons specializing in hand surgery, spine surgery, and sports medicine were included in the hospital's musculoskeletal service line.

The preferential treatment afforded to orthopedic practices created a furor among other physicians on the medical staff, most notably cardiologists and neurosurgeons, who were also interested in preferential treatment of their practices and their service line. If objective guidelines had been adopted, the eventual backlash and acrimonious relationship might have been avoided. Decisions made in the context of overall guidelines will have a higher likelihood of being perceived as fair, objective, and impartial, rather than as targeting one particular physician group unfairly. Of course, adoption of guidelines only increases the likelihood of physician support; it certainly does not guarantee physician buy-in to strategies that influence current and future physician revenue streams, level of physician autonomy, or any real or perceived notions about fair and equal treatment.

SAMPLE GUIDELINES FOR COLLABORATION BETWEEN HOSPITALS AND PHYSICIANS

The following guidelines created for a fictional "General Hospital" help to establish a framework for evaluating potential relationships and opportunities for collaboration as they initially emerge.

- General Hospital will enter into arrangements to share risk and reward through selected joint ventures, joint program development, and other partnerships with physicians whose goals are consistent with those of the hospital.
- Formal partnerships will help position the hospital and medical staff proactively to expand markets and grow services and allow them to share in ambulatory services, as physicians are increasingly motivated to pursue such high-margin services.
- For some services and specific physician practices, competitive strategies will be pursued by the hospital and its medical staff to protect service lines and compete with external initiatives. Such initiatives may include those pursued by the physicians or by independent developers new to the community.
- General Hospital will take a "surgically precise" approach by pursuing alternative partnerships and competitive strategies in which specific initiatives are tailored to particular practices and individual service lines.
- General Hospital will measure and monitor the results of formal partnerships or business relationships to ensure compliance with the original specific, identified objectives of the arrangement and performance targets, including operational, financial, or quality measures.
- General Hospital and its medical staff will focus on a limited number of partnerships (e.g., three or four) each year, in recognition of the high level of effort necessary to accomplish successful implementation and meet potential partnerships' capital requirements.

- The highest priorities for collaboration are those practices and service lines where the hospital and physician partners have the best opportunity to grow and increase market share, the hospital is most vulnerable to outmigration of ancillary services, provision of patient care can be optimized, and financial contributions are (or could be) the highest.
- Physician investment, as demonstrated by significant commitment of effort and personal funds, is essential to help ensure commitment. In similar fashion, hospital leaders who facilitate the formation of formal business relationships should be held personally accountable for the successful implementation of the relationships. Examples of personal accountability include year-end bonuses to compensation, threatened salary cuts, advancement, and the like.
- Preferred relationships will be economic arrangements with private practice(s), as opposed to acquisition or employment of physicians.
- Partnerships will result in a reasonable direct (e.g., financial) and indirect (e.g., improved relationships or goodwill) return on investment or substantially grow the service or program for the hospital and physician practices on the medical staff.

Other guiding principles may be added, or these may be refined, but the preceding guidelines provide a starting point for hospitals and systems that are committed to developing guidelines for establishing stronger, more beneficial relationships through their medical staff organizations.

RATIONALE OR EVALUATION CRITERIA FOR PARTNERSHIPS

In addition to the adoption of general guiding principles, hospitals and their medical staff organizations should develop specific criteria to evaluate individual opportunities for collaboration when they arise. As with the guiding principles, these criteria should be objective and applicable to a variety of situations, opportunities, and initiatives and should be developed when thoughtful and thorough consideration and discussion can occur.

Following are examples of individual evaluation criteria and the questions to ask to determine the criteria. Once the criteria are selected, hospital managers must communicate them broadly to all members of the physician community to avoid being perceived as acting in favoritism to particular segments of the medial staff. In similar fashion, the members of the medical staff organization may want to develop their own evaluation criteria to evaluate their desired position relative to a particular hospital or system.

1. Strategic alignment
- Does the potential partnership further the hospital's mission, vision, and goals? The physician practice's mission, vision, and goals?
- Do hospital leaders and physician practice leaders have a shared vision?
2. Precedent
- Is the partnership likely to set an acceptable precedent for working with any physician practice in a similar arrangement in the future? Alternatively, is the partnership so unique that it will have neither relevance nor applicability to future partnerships? Worse yet, does the partnership establish a bad precedent that may make future similar situations difficult to address?
3. Market position
- Does the hospital-physician partnership in a particular service line improve the quality or outcomes of that particular service, increase volume or market share, or decrease the competitor's market position?
- Additionally, do current and probable future market conditions support the business today, and as it is likely to evolve?
4. Return on investment

- Does the partnership provide adequate return on investment in time, effort, and financial return?
- Does the partnership provide rewards to each party, not to one in a disproportionate manner?

5. The reasonableness of hospital and physician partners
- Are target hospital(s) and physician practice leaders trustworthy, do they have realistic expectations, and are they considerate of each other's goals and concerns?
- Does either partner have a hidden agenda?
- In the planning and development process for the formal partnership, are the planning and negotiation processes—and the information (including goals and objectives)—shared among the participants?

6. Likelihood of threat
- How high is the probability that physicians will develop service independent of the hospital?

7. Magnitude of threat
- Is the potential erosion of hospital ambulatory services volumes, market share, and/or financial threat significant if physicians develop service independent of the hospital?

Applying the Criteria

The application of these criteria can be intriguing and challenging. On the surface, these evaluation criteria can result in specific scores for potential initiatives; however, the relative magnitude of responses is important to consider. To illustrate, consider a scoring system for the evaluation criteria in which a score of -1 indicates a negative score or evaluation for one particular potential partnership, a 0 indicates a neutral score, and a positive result receives a score of $+1$ or $+2$. An example of the application of the evaluation criteria is presented in Figure 7.1.

A particular initiative could receive a score of -10 and another a score of $+20$. The initiative (or initiatives) that score positively are

Figure 7.1. Prioritization Matrix for Possible Physician-Hospital Partnerships

	Partner with For-Profit Orthopedics Hospital	Joint Venture Ambulatory Surgery Centers
Proactive Criteria		
Strategic Alignment	−2	+2
Precedent	0	+1
Market Position	−2	−1
Return on Investment	−1	−1
Reasonable Partners	−2	+2
Reactive Criteria		
Magnitude of Threat	+1	+2
Likelihood of Threat	+1	+1
Consequences	+1	0
TOTAL	−4	+6

Note: Proactive criteria—in anticipation of potential initiative; reactive criteria—in response to initiatives.

Source: Health Strategies & Solutions (2003).

the ones to pursue further, meaning that a detailed business plan for the potential initiative (e.g., joint venture imaging center or ambulatory care center) should be developed. Often a negotiation process, sometimes concurrent with business plan development, follows the identification of priority initiatives.

CONCLUSION

In today's tumultuous environment, physician leaders and hospital managers may have difficulty imagining a roadmap that will lead them out of adversarial and contentious relationships and further separatism between hospitals and physicians. Granted, the path will not be an easy one, but opportunities to develop collaborative working partnerships exist if the medical staff organization is redesigned with a new set of roles and responsibilities tailored to meet the changing needs of both physicians and hospitals.

The medical staff organization of the future will focus on the following six core areas:

1. Improving operations efficiency
2. Contributing to quality improvement
3. Providing economic value for participants
4. Enabling flexibility and evolution
5. Being inclusive, not exclusive
6. Monitoring and evaluating performance

It will be a platform for significant and lasting economic and other partnerships to address the healthcare needs of the communities served. The alternative to revitalizing medical staff organizations is further exacerbation of competition and independence that in the long run will not serve communities well, is detrimental to physicians and hospitals, and will waste valuable healthcare resources.

These lofty goals will be accomplished by creative, individually tailored strategies that make the eventual partnership arrangements much more challenging, yet more lasting. Difficult challenges and major opportunities line the long road toward collaborative efforts to create the successful medical staff organization of the future.

REFERENCES

Afable, R. 2003. Personal interview, July 28.

Health Strategies & Solutions. 2003. Various materials.

About the Author

Craig E. Holm, CHE, is a founding partner and director at Health Strategies & Solutions, Inc., a leading independent healthcare management consulting firm based in Philadelphia. Mr. Holm's practice focuses on strategy development for physicians, hospitals, and health systems. He has been a management consultant since 1984. He previously served as a hospital administrator at Strong Memorial Hospital in 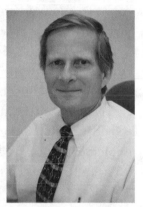 Rochester, New York, and at Clifton Springs Hospital in Clifton Springs, New York.

Mr. Holm earned his undergraduate degree and a master's degree in business administration from Cornell University. He is a diplomate of the American College of Healthcare Executives and a member of the American Association of Healthcare Consultants. Mr. Holm is published widely and is a frequent speaker for national healthcare conferences. His first book, *Next Generation Physician–Health System Partnerships*, was published by Health Administration Press in 2000.

Mr. Holm lives in suburban Philadephia with his wife, Karen, and children Shannon, Spencer, and Connor.

About the Contributors

Richard F. Afable, M.D., is executive vice president and chief medical officer of Catholic Health East (CHE), one of the largest healthcare systems in the United States with 32 acute care hospitals and 27 long-term-care facilities. He is responsible for the system's clinical performance, quality of care, cost-reduction initiatives, and managed care coordination. Prior to joining CHE in 1999, Dr. Afable was the founder and president/chief executive officer of Preferred Physician Partners, LLC, a provider resource company that supports physician groups and provider networks in managed care markets.

Dr. Afable has more than 20 years of medical practice experience as a solo practitioner and in small group and academic group practice. He has served as an associate professor of medicine at Wake Forest University Bowman Gray School of Medicine and as clinical assistant professor at Feinberg School of Medicine, Northwestern University. Dr. Afable has led numerous consulting engagements, including network development, PSO development, provider profiling and reporting, information system design and implementation, medical management development and execution, and physician leadership programs. He is a fellow of the American College of Physicians.

Russell C. Coile, Jr., is the late editor of *Russ Coile's Health Trends* and was senior strategist for Health Strategies & Solutions, a healthcare consulting firm based in Philadelphia. He was a nationally recognized futurist who provided market forecasts and strategic advice to hospitals, medical groups, health plans, and suppliers on a nationwide basis. In 2002, he was ranked among the "top 100 health leaders" by *Modern Healthcare* magazine.

Mr. Coile was the author of ten books and numerous articles on the future of the health field. Since 2001, Mr. Coile participated in more than 100 seminars for groups including the American Hospital Association, the American College of Healthcare Executives, the

Governance Institute, the American College of Physician Executives, and the Health Information and Management Systems Society.

Mr. Coile was the past president of the Society for Healthcare Strategy and Market Development of the American Hospital Association and a board member of the Center for Health Design and the Public Health Institute. He was also a member of editorial advisory boards, including *Managed Care Outlook*, *Nurse Week*, and *Healthcare Market Strategist*. Mr. Coile passed away in November 2003.

Hugo J. Finarelli, Jr., Ph.D., is a recognized expert in quantitative analysis and demand forecasting, with more than 30 years of systems analysis and hospital planning experience. He is a founding partner and director of Health Strategies & Solutions, Inc., a leading national healthcare consulting firm based in Philadelphia. Dr. Finarelli directs the firm's data activities, specializing in the development of customized computer models and population-based demand forecasts.

He was formerly vice president of two other healthcare consulting firms and has also held positions with firms specializing in public policy issues and regional healthcare planning. Dr. Finarelli has a master's degree in mathematics from the Massachusetts Institute of Technology and a doctorate in systems engineering and operations research from the University of Pennsylvania.